"The author discusses the challenges facing a psychoanalysis that refuses to be a relic. Tesone re-thinks subjective production through the vicissitudes of the drives and their identification destiny, in a trajectory from indiscrimination to the acceptance of otherness and subjective evolution. How can we produce theoretical thinking anchored in clinical experience and capable of fighting dogmatism? How do we consider the complexity of the subject, which oscillates between the redundant and the unpredictable, between repetition and novelty? These questions permeate his book. It provokes enthusiasm because it dares to be open while also based on experience. A book that invites a dialogue. It has brought me to re-think notions I thought definitive. For this I am grateful and recommend it."

—**Dr. Luis Horstein,** *physician and psychoanalyst,*
President of FUNDEP (Foundation for Psychoanalytic Studies)

"The author highlights two poles that structure the traumatic: the existence of the other and the subject's own sexuality. He emphasizes the specific in what is Disruptive, the Traumatic, and Symbolization: a total lack of representation, a black hole of the psyche. He alerts us to the excess of binding as the antithesis of chaos, which is the basis of psychic change. In this sense, psychoanalysis is called upon to work through the tension between the sexes of the phallic order and the 'nothing' order, generating idiosyncratic representations and overcoming the cisgender product of thwarting binarism. In this set of psychoanalytic texts, Tesone gives us a creative, in-depth discussion of the vicissitudes of the body."

—**Moty Benyakar**, *physician, psychiatrist, and Full*
Member of the Israeli Psychoanalytic Society; Professor
Emeritus of the USAL, M.D., Ph.D., Director of the Contem-
porary Psychoanalysis and the Disruptive Committee in the
doctoral program in Psychology of the USAL; Full Member
of the Argentine Psychoanalytic Association and of the
International Psychoanalytical Association

Trauma and Pain Without a Subject

Trauma and Pain Without a Subject explores the necessity of the subject of trauma emerging, particularly when a victim has experienced but not worked through disruptive situations, in order for unconscious pain to finally be experienced.

The book is presented in three parts, with the first, "Transgression and Crime", uncovering silence around the topic of incest and sexual violence within the clinic. The second part, "Between Completeness and Nothingness", develops the topic of sexual violence and considers the construction of femininities and masculinities within the paradigm of a heteronormative patriarchal society, with reference to Shakespeare's *Much Ado About Nothing*. The third part, "Yes, We See, But What? What We Hear", explores the intimate relation between the visual and the auditory, especially in relation to hysteria.

Trauma and Pain Without a Subject will be of great interest to psychoanalysts in practice and in training, and to all psychoanalytic practitioners working with trauma.

Juan-Eduardo Tesone is Emeritus Professor of Psychoanalysis at the University of Salvador (USAL), Argentina, and Associate Professor of Psychology at Paris Nanterre University, France. He is a Member and Training Analyst of the Argentine Psychoanalytic Association and Member of the International Psychoanalytical Association. He is the author of more than 100 articles in specialist journals, in Spanish, French, English, Italian, German, Portuguese, and Croatian, and author and co-author of several books.

Psychoanalytic Ideas and Applications Series

Series Editor: Silvia Flechner
IPA Publications Committee
Natacha Delgado, Nergis Güleç, Thomas Marcacci, Carlos Moguillansky,
Rafael Mondrzak, Angela M. Vuotto, Gabriela Legoretta (consultant)

Recent titles in the Series include

The Infinite Infantile and the Psychoanalytic Task
Psychoanalysis with Children, Adolescents and their Families
*Edited by Nilde Parada Franch, Christine Anzieu-Premmereur,
Mónica Cardenal and Majlis Winberg Salomonsson*

A Psychoanalytic Understanding of Trauma
Post-Traumatic Mental Functioning, the Zero Process,
and the Construction of Reality
Joseph Fernando

The Poetry of the Word in Psychoanalysis
Selected Papers of Pere Folch Mateu
Edited by J.O. Esteve and Jordi Sala

The Freudian Matrix of André Green
Towards a Psychoanalysis for the 21st Century
Edited by Howard B. Levine

Desire, Pain and Thought
Primal Masochism and Psychoanalytic Theory
Marilia Aisenstein

Trauma and Pain Without a Subject
Disruptive Marks in the Psyche, Resignified
Juan-Eduardo Tesone

For more information about this series, please visit: www.routledge.com

Trauma and Pain Without a Subject

Disruptive Marks in the Psyche, Resignified

Juan-Eduardo Tesone

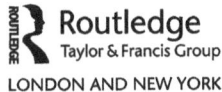
Routledge
Taylor & Francis Group

LONDON AND NEW YORK

Designed cover image: Getty | fcscafeine

First published 2024
by Routledge
4 Park Square, Milton Park, Abingdon, Oxon OX14 4RN

and by Routledge
605 Third Avenue, New York, NY 10158

Routledge is an imprint of the Taylor & Francis Group, an informa business

© 2024 Juan-Eduardo Tesone

British Library Cataloguing-in-Publication Data
A catalogue record for this book is available from the British Library

ISBN: 978-1-032-64778-4 (hbk)
ISBN: 978-1-032-64777-7 (pbk)
ISBN: 978-1-032-64779-1 (ebk)

DOI: 10.4324/9781032647791

Typeset in Palatino
by codeMantra

Contents

About the author

Juan-Eduardo Tesone, MD, PhD, is Emeritus Professor of Psychoanalysis at the University of Salvador (USAL), Argentina, and Associate Professor of Psychology at Paris Nanterre University, France. He received his degree as a psychiatrist from Paris XII University. He did his analyst training and became Full Member of the Paris Psychoanalytical Society (1992–2019). He is a Full Member and Training Analyst of the Argentine Psychoanalytic Association and a Member of the International Psychoanalytical Association. For eleven years he directed a center for psychotherapy (Centre-Médico-Psycho-Pédagogique Pichon-Riv-ière), in connection with Juvenile Justice in Paris, which specialized in the subject of physical and/or sexual violence towards minors. He also directed "SOS Family in Danger", a telephone counseling center for potentially violent parents who wished to seek help. He is the author of more than 100 articles in specialist journals, in Spanish, French, English, Italian, German, Portuguese, and Croatian; co-author of 18 books in various languages; and author of *In the Traces of Our Name: The Influence of Given Names in Life*, which was given an award by the Ministry of Culture of the Argentine Nation (2011) and also, in 2019, by the IPA, which gave the book its most important award granted by it for a psychoanalytic work. He has been bestowed Chevalier de l'Ordre National du Mérite (2013) and Chevalier des Palmes Académiques (2021) by thet French Government.

Series editor's foreword

The Publications Committee of the International Psychoanalytical Association presents a new volume in the series "Psychoanalytic Ideas and Applications".

The aim of this series is to focus on the scientific production of significant authors whose works are outstanding contributions to the psychoanalytic field and to set out relevant ideas and themes generated during the history of psychoanalysis, that deserve to be known and discussed by psychoanalysts of our Association.

Our goal is to share these ideas with the psychoanalytic community and professionals of related disciplines, to expand their knowledge and generate a productive interchange between the text and the reader. The IPA Publications Committee is pleased to publish Juan-Eduardo Tessone's book *A pain without a subject.*

Dr. Juan-Eduardo Tesone is a member of the International Psychoanalytic Association, Full Member of the Argentine Psychoanalytic Association (APA), and former Member of the Paris Psychoanalytical Society (SPP)

This book is composed of three parts. The first, titled "Transgression and Crime", concerns a relatively taboo problem: incest. Dr. Tesone argues that hearing about Oedipus in psychoanalysis is much more frequent, but one rarely hears about consummated incest. He states that incest is not more intense than Oedipus. On the contrary, it is the denial of incest. Oedipus builds subjectivity by enabling acceptance of lack, whereas incest destroys any otherness and, consequently, the child's subjectivity.

Dr. Tesone tries to deepen transdisciplinary dialogue with Law, Philosophy, Linguistics, Semiology, and Anthropology through his theorization. In this endeavor, he takes psychoanalytic practice out of the abbey of the consulting room and into a position in community mental health.

The second part is titled "Between Completeness and Nothingness". The subject of completeness is futilely sought by all human beings when confronted with nothingness, but it is historically attributed to women by a hetero-normative patriarchal perspective. For the author, nothingness in the form of symbolic castration concerns every human being, independent of sex or gender. William Shakespeare contributes to his proposal through *Much Ado About Nothing*.

In chapter 16, "Cumulative Trauma and 'troumatique'", he interrogates the field of traumatic questions in a paradigmatic way: the unrepresentable, putting in tension the classic analytic device of making the unconscious conscious, revealing that in this clinic, the lifting of repression is not enough to trace something unconsciously to become a mnemic trace. On the contrary, on certain occasions the traumatic experience generates a vacuum of figuration that aspires to every possible form of representation.

Finally, the author cites Borges, the great clinician of the human soul who has left, in *The Aleph* (1949), a particularly hope-inspiring sentence for our clinical work: "To change the past is not to change a mere single event; it is to annul all its consequences, which tend to infinity." Likewise, the French poet Paul Valéry summarizes: "The past has a future." The author agrees with both writers and allows himself to add that when the past is no longer mere repetition, something new and creative may emerge.

For the author, "the red thread that runs through this book is the disruptive marks, in filigree in any disruptive condition, that, to the extent that they can be resignified, will allow the elaboration of the traumatic feeling.

Silvia Flechner
Series Editor
Chair, IPA Publications Committee

Preface

In order to write the introduction to a book, it is necessary to generate interest and enthusiasm. It also needs to have a connection with the text in order to show that it does not necessarily imply theoretical agreement with the author. Even so, it also needs to generate excitement that spontaneously creates desire to discuss ideas. Having been given all three circumstances, I think Juan treasured his invitation to write this short text, which honors me. From the introduction, Juan's book generates a state of expectation by beginning to explain the reason for his writing. Juan refers to this as an aid to process the experiences that occurred in the analytic sessions from the past until what happened in the moment. It also refers to the self-therapeutic value for psychoanalysts, who write by allowing themselves to process both the patient's suffering as their own. There he thinks that instead of transference and countertransference, he prefers to call it a reciprocal transference. It is very striking when Juan refers to this double condition as a sedentary lifestyle in relation to the recurring themes; the different cultures he has inhabited throughout his life and with some nomadism in the geographical sense. It is during this time period that we have shared some special moments of our lives.

Juan was born in Buenos Aires, but grew up in Mar del Plata, a city 400 km south of the capital. After high school, he went to study Medicine at the University of Buenos Aires, and that was where we met for the first time in our fourth year, in the hospital, where we both attended from Monday to Saturday. The hospital unit was a melting pot of knowledge about ailments, both physical and psychical. During this period, our sensitivity was tested. They were three years of great awareness and in contact with the suffering of human beings. We were very young, and we enjoyed it very much. It was medicine up close and real, which we had not observed before and which left its mark. I remember the reaction when I told my group of friends at the end of my studies that I had decided to dedicate myself to psychoanalysis. They appeared to be sad as they rested their hands on my shoulder. It seemed that maybe I had forgotten about the body and real medicine. It felt that they had lost someone. I never asked Juan how his process was, but I suspect it was similar. Afterwards we were companions for a brief time on a course in psychotherapy for children. Shortly after that, Juan left for Paris. At this moment in time, 1978, I had two very young children, so I stayed and began analytic training. Many years later, Juan and I would meet again in various congresses throughout Europe. We found ourselves among the climate of nomadism of psychoanalysts which does not only include those who have lived for many years outside their country.

On Juan's return to Argentina, we got in touch again and so we continue our friendship. We both know that the thread "invisible to the eye" that unites and sustains us is always there.

I will now return to Juan's introduction. There the author poses a question that opens new paths to think about language: Your experience of living in two cultures with two different languages?

This has led Juan to consider the way in which language and subjectivities undoubtedly impact our way of thinking when shifting from one language to another, in his case Spanish and French. This has multiplied the senses and also has the freedom of movement between different psychoanalytic theories. Jacques Derrida goes so far as to say that a psychoanalyst should speak at least two different languages.

This book is divided into three parts that bring together and, in turn, develop three themes: In the first, entitled "Transgression and Crime", it addresses a theme of hot news, such as sexual abuse with implied violence. Juan cites that fact and also the question of incest. He also draws our attention to how little psychoanalytic literature there is in relation to consummated incest. He proposes that this issue has been condemned in the psychoanalytic clinic to the same silence as that of the victim of consummated incest. This observation, together with the development he makes on the subject in dialogue with other disciplines, opens a path that exhorts us to continue thinking. He also gives voice to what happens to ourselves when we are confronted with these stories in our consultation rooms.

In the second part, "Between Completeness and Nothingness", Juan continues developing the issue of sexual violence, which he prefers to "sexual abuse". He then ventures into current topics of debate, which also imply the construction of femininities and masculinities within the paradigm of patriarchal society. This part also includes a very interesting chapter on tattooing which is illustrated by clinical material. In addition, it shows us that the clinical psychoanalyst has great experience in the analysis of children and adolescents.

In the third part, which bears as its title a phrase of the French poet, Jacques Ancet: "Yes, We See, But What? What We Hear." This studies the relationship between what one sees and what is heard starting from hysteria. The developments of this part of the volume are particularly interesting and contribute to dissolving a debate on the importance of observation over listening or vice versa, a discussion at this point, as well as the author, I consider it obsolete. It is known that for the British School of

Psychoanalysis, the notion of unconscious fantasy is tinged with a strong accent on the perceptual–visual. The tradition of French psychoanalysis, moreover, coherent with the notion of structure and the Lacanian concept of the unconscious structured as a language, gets along better with the analyst's focus located in listening. Even so, it is true that as soon as we approach the clinic, this polarization will be difficult to sustain: An analyst who "listens" to his patient does not register music, tone of voice, or body language, nor noises from outside the office, or their own bodily thoughts and sensations?

Lastly, and to let readers begin their own journey in this exciting volume, I found its title to be a discovery. From the reading of the different chapters, it emerges in a kind of *après-coup*, the notion that violence, in this case sexual, is desubjective, destroys the possibility of going through the necessary processes of subjectivation, and much more in childhood, puberty, and adolescence. The processes have been disruptive, I would say lacerating of the tissue necessary for the Self, even to experience pain. Hence, the great value and the great commitment of the psychoanalyst are to offer a space for historicism and also for the opportunity of subjectivation. Only then, when there is a subject, will he or she be able to feel the pain.

This is a book that is just as important and necessary in a world like the one we have today. We are now living after a pandemic, which has forced us to live with uncertainty and also with violence in its various forms. Even the horror of a war compels us to think and talk, to give voice to all those who do not have it. Finally, even Freud, so criticized for his position in relation to women, gave them a voice when he invited his first patients to associate freely on his couch, in what he called the "Talking Cure."

Virginia Ungar
Past President of the IPA and Full Member of APdeBA
(Buenos Aires Psychoanalytical Associations)
Buenos Aires, November 2022

Introduction

As psychoanalysts, we may feel the need to write for more than one reason. First: we need to consider our working through of the clinical relation with our patients; second: it is a medium for thinking outside the urgency of the session and reflecting on what was said. Third, and at the same time, it is a way to be close to our patients while also preserving the distance we need to think about their complex problems. No less important: a way to find adequate proximity and distance between the other's conflicts and our own, given that writing is an effort to work through the anxieties of clinical practice whose obstacles stimulated Freudian theorization.

Writing may calm anxieties and make it possible for clinical work, confronted with suffering, to work through, digest, and return it to our patients, metabolized, whether by pointing out, interpreting, or constructing something that brings relief to the suffering, both the patient's and the analyst's. "Transference" and "countertransference" are the terms commonly used, but I prefer the idea of reciprocal transference.

I was encouraged to gather my earlier writings for this book, whereby I discovered internal cohesion in lectures I had given in different places and articles I had published in journals in different languages. This quiescence, so to speak, of themes I found to recur in diverse cultures, and it contrasts with the geographical nomadism that has enriched my adult life.

I lived in Argentina in Mar del Plata during my childhood and adolescence, a city by the sea whose perpetual movement defined my perception of the real; the maritime horizon inspiring a wish to reach beyond that imaginary line. I studied medicine at the University of Buenos Aires and specialized in psychopathology at the "Ricardo Gutierrez" Children's Hospital, also in Buenos Aires. Formative years were, I would say, followed by a lifetime of "days of ongoing training." A scholarship and a local *coup d'état* sent me to France in 1976, where I lived for 22 years.

I worked in Paris as a psychiatrist at the "La Salpêtrière" Hospital; I trained as a psychoanalyst at the Paris Psychoanalytical Society and "L'École Freudienne"; I was the director of a center for ambulatory psychotherapy for children and adolescents, which, at my suggestion, is named after the great Franco-Argentine professor, Enrique Pichon-Rivière. I held

DOI: 10.4324/9781032647791-1

a post as Associate Professor at the University of Paris-Nanterre, where I received my doctorate in psychology. Later, on my return to Buenos Aires in 1998, I became a Member of the Argentine Psychoanalytic Association, and I continue to teach at several Argentine and foreign universities, in particular as Professor Emeritus in the doctoral program, "The Disruptive and Psychoanalysis" at Salvador University, chaired by Professor Moty Benyakar. I work and study in both my languages.

My confrontation with a different culture, but especially with a different language, led me to be doubly aware of language: on the one hand, the way it determines our way of thinking. Some of these texts were written in Spanish; others were written in French and later translated into Spanish. It is striking to note how the passage from one language to another multiplies meanings, semantics, and also perceptions of the real world. This duality generates enough stimuli for me to feel I am not inscribed in any one place or language or to any one theory as a reference. On the other hand, I have found a red thread that runs through cultures, languages, theories, and disciplines, stringing together my texts through years and geographies.

I propose the reading of this book in its three parts.

Part I is entitled "Transgression and Crime." Its major themes concern a problem that is relatively taboo: that of incest. In psychoanalysis, we frequently hear about the Oedipus, but rarely about consummated incest. Incest is not a more intense Oedipus. On the contrary, it is the denial of incest. The Oedipus builds subjectivity by enabling acceptance of lack, whereas incest destroys any kind of otherness and consequently the child's subjectivity.

Through my theorization I aim to deepen transdisciplinary dialogue with Law, Philosophy, Linguistics, Semiology, and Anthropology. In this endeavor, I take psychoanalytic practice out of the cloister of the consulting room and into a position in community mental health.

Especially concerning the latter, I describe the contributions of Claude Lévi-Strauss and Françoise Héritier regarding the characteristics of the taboo against incest. I draw a distinction between what is different and what is identical, and also examine ways to ontologically clarify issues of gender, sex, parentality, and alliance, revealing the pact of restriction and the system of regulation in culture. Steering the course into disruptive scars, some ancestral myths about incest are dismantled, and, to exemplify, I conjugate aspects of clinical practice relating to the abject in the family scene and its sinister implications.

Part II, "Between Completeness and Nothingness," covers the subject of completeness futilely sought by all human beings when confronted with nothingness but historically attributed to women by a hetero-normative patriarchal perspective. Nothingness in the form of symbolic castration concerns every human being, independent of sex and/or gender. William Shakespeare contributes to my concept through *Much Ado About Nothing*. When Shakespeare wrote this play, in 1600, in the form of a comedy, a Renaissance conception of women was placed in tension. His text distills subtle irony regarding prejudices about women and men in his time. On the lips of Beatrice he sets incisive and provocative dialogue with Benedict in a duel between equal, unusual for his era; they both deny love, but in the end become spouses. Through Hero, the daughter of Leonato, all of men's fears concerning women's infidelity appear, as well as the seal of disapproval reserved for women if they are not virgins when they marry. We may assume that this play is a satire on the condition of women and that it was not worth making such "ado" about Hero's allegedly missing virginity or her false infidelity. However, "nothing" in Elizabethan slang means vagina. Therefore, "nothing" was intended to mean that women had nothing (no-thing) between their legs. In this point of view, Freud's dark continent would be an expression of the unexplored and the enigmatic, but also of complexity exceeding the phallic register. I discuss this term *nothing* in greater detail in Chapter 13.

In the "Divine Jouissance, the Feminine Position, and the Mystics" (chapter 10) I consider feminine pleasure. Through centuries of male domination, female enjoyment has not been readily admitted —a prohibition of which hysterics were the main victims. They were the victims of such intolerance, paying a heavy price, sometimes at the cost of their own lives at the stake of the Inquisition. Even today, mutilation-excision of the clitoris is practiced on girls in vast areas of the world, condemning women to not obtaining the pleasure that this organ normally gives them.

What if the discourse of the mystics showed, in an extreme way although veiled by religious demands, the additional enjoyment of women, otherwise unspeakable if one does not want to suffer the same punishment as Tiresias?

The title of Part III quotes a fragment by the French poet, Jacques Ancet, suggesting the intimate relation between the visual and the auditory, especially in relation to hysteria: "Yes, We See, But What? What We Hear."

To analyze is to analyze discourse, the language the person is made of, its anchor points and points of "*capitonné*," and also the affects running through both tongues and silences. Although remembering and infantile amnesia are classically valued for their subversion of repression, the need to forget has not been adequately considered —not just any forgetting, but forgetting that, as in mourning, enables decatechization of the object of grief. The short story, "Funes the Memorious", by Jorge Luis Borges (1944), is an eloquent example of the need of a certain kind of forgetting that enables thinking. The psychic apparatus functions as a sort of conflictive alchemy between remembering and forgetting. Both are necessary to preserve a sense of identity and the ability to think—an eternal oscillation between memory's imagination and the creative ability to forget.

In chapter 16, "Cumulative Trauma and '*Troumatique*'," we examine in a paradigmatic way the field of the traumatic question—the unrepresentable— putting in tension the classic analytic device of making the unconscious conscious and revealing that in this clinic the lifting of repression is not enough for tracing something anemic to become mnemic. The traumatic experience in the analytic session generates, at times, a vacuum of figuration that aspires to every possible form of representation. What inscription does the perception of the disruptive fact acquire? Regarding this question, my purpose will be to open a path rather than indicate an itinerary. Why do I call this book *Trauma and Pain Without a Subject*? Because it is often necessary for the subject to emerge, particularly when a victim has experienced disruptive situations but not worked them through, in order for a pain encysted in the unconscious, outside the circulation of signifiers, to finally be experienced. The discourse of trauma, one must point out, is always carried by someone desubjectivized by knowledge inscribed in the body, to the point that it suspends both judging attributions as well as judging existence. When time is stopped, it is because a subject is needed in order to have time, and in order to have a subject and, therefore, repression, a succession of signifiers is necessary. In the case of trauma, the chain of signifiers is interrupted, and it is precisely at this place that time is stopped, awaiting a new signifier.

Cloistered by a supposedly protective membrane, this pain undermines subjectivity. Only when the subject is able to appear, associated with the pain, when the membrane of this black hole sucking subjectivity into it becomes porous, its potentially traumatic scars entering circulation and being worked through, can the subject reappear and experience that pain resignified; this is the only way to metabolize it; the only means for a split-off pain to finally become suffering inhabited by a subject who accepts it as their own; it takes internal time rather than linear or calendar time.

I proposed above that the reader follow the order suggested by the succession of parts, progressively threading together the concepts in the chain of ideas. However, each chapter may also be read independently, in the context of the particular interests it may awaken in the reader. Since I tend to prefer a plurality of approaches, I do not imagine I have found all the possible meanings in the chain of the real. Perhaps what is most genuine is the existential value its writing has acquired for me and the pleasure of sharing it.

Last but not least, Borges, the great clinician of the human soul, has left us, in "The Aleph" (1949), a particularly hope-inspiring sentence for our clinical work: "To change the past is not to change a mere single event; it is to annul all its consequences, which tend to infinity." The French poet Paul Valéry summarizes: "The past has a future." I agree with both writers, and allow myself to add: when the past is no longer mere repetition, something new and creative may emerge.

The red thread that runs throughout this book is the disruptive marks, in filigree in any disruptive condition, that, to the extent that they can be resignified, will allow the elaboration of the traumatic feeling.

References

Borges, J. L. (1944). Funes el Memorioso [Funes the Memorious]. In: *Obras Completas* (pp. 483–485). Buenos Aires: Emecé, 1974.

Borges, J. L. (1949). El Aleph. In: *Obras completas* (p. 573). Buenos Aires: Emecé, 1974.

Part I
Transgression and crime

1 Incests and transgression of the narcissistic taboo*

The term "incest" is derived from the Latin *in-cestus*, which means un-chaste, impure; its antonym, *castus*, refers to what is pure, unsullied, but especially, in terms of the rites and rules, proper.

Although we commonly speak of "incest," I think the term should be used in the plural, given the variability it presents in the diverse fields that discuss it from anthropological, legal, or psychoanalytic perspectives. Incest, or rather incests, provokes horror and fascination, repulsion and attraction, generating the emotional intensity that probably induced the circumstance that this complex problem has not been thought about: it has, instead, been sealed, at least in clinical work, into the same silence that is forced upon the victims. In recent years, it has returned via the mass media, but in a sensationalistic way, where it is reported frequently, but not always adequately. When we review psychoanalytic literature, we are surprised to find that few texts refer to consummated incest. Beyond Freud's writings, which mention it, especially in Totem and Taboo (1912), contemporary psychoanalytic literature has published texts on it only in the last two decades. It is deplorable that a problem associated with humankind since ancient times, described in the Bible, mythology, literature, and anthropology, has not found an echo equal to its importance in the psychoanalytic field. Psychoanalysis discusses incestuous wishes quite easily, but not consummated incests. To what point has psychoanalysis become fixated on Freud's abandonment of what he considered "his neurotics" (Freud, 1898)? We know that he renounced them only partially, and that near the end of his life he admitted the frequent existence of real scenes of seduction with severe pathological impact.

However, we need first to ask what it is that provokes its prohibition. The laws in many countries consider sexual abuse aggravated when the perpetrator is a close older relative and the victim is underage. However,

* This is an expanded and modified version of my article, "Los incestos y la negación de la alteridad" ["Incests and the negation of otherness"], in Revista de Psicoanálisis (Buenos Aires), Vol. 61, No. 4, 2004.

DOI: 10.4324/9781032647791-3

the penal code does not use the term "incest." The French penal code introduced this term only quite recently. The penal code in many other countries does not consider incestuous relations between adults a crime. Although the civil code regulates the degree of kinship that allows marriage, it does not regulate sexual relations between others that may be incestuous.

Anthropology is the field that has thought the most about the prohibition of incest and has elaborated theories on it. Here again, we need to ask what it is that provokes its prohibition. We review the anthropological perspective, since psychoanalysis may share a certain view, although the reasons for the prohibition may not be isomorphic, and psychoanalysts may approach the need of prohibition via different though confluent paths.

Why do we prohibit incest?

In his book, *The Origin of the Family, Private Property and the State* (1884), Engels assumed that in prehistoric times the family lived in such promiscuity that sexual relations existed between all its members. This family modality, according to Engels, soon disappeared and was replaced by family groups before the formation of the contemporary family. We may ask: at the beginning, was there absolute disorder? Nothing is more uncertain in Engels' thesis. Modern anthropological theories agree in denying the existence, even in earliest times, of such family magma.

In *Totem and Taboo* (1912–13), Freud proposed to explain the prohibition of incest through the repentance of the brothers following parricide and their alliance as a mechanism to regulate social relations.

In spite of the anthropological uncertainty of this myth, it has the advantage, as Lévi-Strauss (1947) believed, of successfully explaining the dawn of civilization.

This French author made the prohibition of incest the paradigm of his theorization, highlighting its universality. It is the primacy of exogamic law over endogamy, based on giving away and the rule of reciprocity.

However, as Lacan (1959) points out, although Lévi-Strauss indicates why the father does not marry his daughter (daughters must be exchanged), he does not say why the son does not have sexual relations with his mother.

Incest as defined by Lévi-Strauss is extended by F. Héritier (1994), who adds a different type of incest, with heavy anthropological and clinical implications: she calls it the "second type," to differentiate it from the Lévi-Straussian "first type." She conceives of the prohibition of incest as a problem of the circulation of fluids from one body to another. According to this anthropologist, the basic criterion of incest is the contact between identical humors, which involves the most fundamental element of human society: its mode of constructing categories of the identical and the different. Héritier (1994, p. 12) states that "The prohibition of incest protects from the horror of the identical." You may not "put the same onto the same," explain the Samo people, who use the term "the dog's way" to designate incest.

The "second type" of incest is indirect incest, which unites two close blood relations through a common sexual partner. I review the theory of this anthropologist because Lévi-Straussian incest does not explain the prohibition in certain communities against a man having sexual relations with his first wife's sister. It includes several variants, such as a man with two sisters, a man with his wife's daughter (identity of substance between mother and daughter) or, symmetrically, a woman with two brothers, a woman with her husband's son, etc. All these incests assume the meeting of humors between two identical fleshes through a common partner. The incest takes place through another person by way of "humors," the body substances that travel from one to the other by means of their transitive character through a body shared at successive times.

This author proposes a reinterpretation of incest in Sophocles' tragedy: does Oedipus, in the depths of the sexual encounter with his mother, also find his father, who was there before him? This homosexual variant has heavy clinical impact in psychoanalysis.

Héritier finds that prohibitions are not explained simply by the rule of marriage division that enables construction of the social bond as defined by Lévi-Strauss. She introduces what she considers most fundamental in human societies: "the way they construct their categories of the identical and the different" (Héritier, 1994) The opposition between the identical and the different is the first category, according to Héritier. She considers incest an accumulation of the identical: "these crimes have traits in common: they fail to separate what must be separated, mix what must be kept apart, and confuse genders, sexes, parentality, and alliance."

I consider that this difficulty in conceiving the qualities of difference and otherness occupies thecenter of the clinical problem of the incestuous act. It is related to narcissistic pathology.

Depending on the culture, consummated incest, which accumulates the identical, may be considered to provoke natural catastrophes such as hurricanes, floods, droughts, etc.—an indivisible association between symbolic human disorder and the way of nature.

However, the prohibition of incest is not simply a prohibition: while it prohibits, it also provides order. To underscore this ordering aspect, I propose to examine an imaginary initial interview in which the patient tells his future psychoanalyst his reason for consulting:

A psychoanalyst receives a young adult for an initial interview, and asks what has brought him to consult. The future patient answers, "Well, everything started when I got married. I made a huge mistake! I married a widow who had a 25-year-old daughter, who became my step-daughter. One day, my father visits us and, incredibly, falls in love with my step-daughter. Shortly afterwards, my father and my step-daughter get married. Suddenly, my step-daughter becomes my step-mother. Sometime after that, my wife and I have a son who becomes my father's brother-in-law, since he is my step-daughter's half-brother and she is my father's wife (and therefore my step-mother). Now, my baby is also my step-mother's half-brother and therefore is a bit my uncle. My wife is also my step-grand-mother, since she is my step-mother's mother. And don't forget that my step-mother is also my step-daughter. And if we look a bit further, we see that I'm my step-grandmother's husband, and therefore I'm not only my wife's grandson and also her husband, but I'm also my own grandfather. Do you understand why I came to see you?

The fictional humor of this interview reminds me that the family creates and institutes three relational orders: (1) consanguinity (brother, sister); (2) alliance (the couple); and (3) filiation (son, daughter).

In this sense, it is an institution, since it institutes an order. Each person occupies a position assigned by the structure. The existence of the family intrinsically and always assumes an order that enables others to recognize who is who or, in other words, each individual's position. As underscored by M. C. and E. Ortigues (1966), nobody may say who is who without making a certain number of choices between the logical possibilities offered by language to allude to positional value: a person is a son or daughter, father or mother, brother or sister, etc. The prohibition of incest supports a logical function without which everything would become obscure, confusing each person's limits.

Benveniste (1969) studies the evolution of different kinship terms in the Indo-European languages and explains their classificatory function. He points out the greater importance of the function over the blood relation, which may or may not exist. The value of the kinship term is given by its position in the family structure. The value of each position is representational rather than absolute. Beyond the place given by biology, we are led to consider the symbolic function exerted depending on the position occupied. What is important about the possibility of parentality is not the position of the biological genitor but rather this person's capacity to carry out that symbolic function of parentality. This function may or may not correspond to biological filiation. Therefore, we could say that all maternity or paternity is, by definition, adoptive, since it requires recognition of the other and recognition of oneself as a link in a chain of trans generational symbolic functions. A child requires a symbolic family order in order to emerge as a subject. This order presumes a difference between the generations.

The *princeps* function of the family, whatever form it may take, is to produce otherness (Tesone, 2004). Transgression of the prohibition in the family consists, according to R. Barthes (1971), in altering the terminological clarity of the parental profile that produces a single signified. An example is the girl named Olympia in de Sade's novel, who is given various simultaneous names. Olympia, says de Sade's incestuous monk, "unites the triple honour of being my daughter, my granddaughter, and my niece." "The transgression lies in naming outside the lexical division," according to Barthes; transgression in this perspective is seen as a surprise of naming. This author highlights that incest consists in transgressing a semantic rule by creating a homonymy, that is to say, incest is also a surprise in vocabulary.

References

Barthes, R. (1971). *Sade, Fourier, Loyola*. Paris: Seuil,

Benveniste, E. (1969). *Le vocabulaire des institutions Indo-Européennes*. Paris: Editions de Minuit.

Engels (1884). *El origen de la familia. La propiedad privada y el Estado* [The origin of the family, private property and the state]. Moscú: Editorial Progreso, 1966.

Freud, S. (1898). Sexuality in the aetiology of the neurosies. In: *Standard Edition, Vol. 3*. London: Hogarth Press, 1953.

Freud, S. (1912–13). *Totem and Taboo*.In: *Standard Edition, Vol. 13*. London: Hogarth Press, 1953.

Héritier, F. (1994). *Les deux soeurs et leur mère*. Paris: Editions Odile Jacob.

Lacan, J. (1959). Das ding. In: *Le séminaire, Livre VII*. Paris: Seuil, 1986.

Lévi-Strauss, C. (1947). Les principes de la parenté. In: *Les structures élémentaires de la parenté*. Paris: Mouton, 1967.

Ortigues, M. C., & Ortigues, E. (1966). *L'oedipe africain*. Paris: Plon.

Sade, Marquis de (1994). *Justine ou les malheurs de la vertu*. Paris: Gallimard.

Tesone, J.-E. (2004). Los incestos y la negación de la alteridad. *Revista de Psicoanálisis, Buenos Aires, 61* (4): 857–878.

2   Incest is not the Oedipus

Beyond the horror, not without fascination, produced by the transgression of humanity's oldest taboo, how do we think about the unthinkable? It is difficult to accept that what we on the outside would label as abject and ignominious is often found in a particular type of naturalized family, almost as a style of communication that sometimes goes on for years; everybody knows about it and yet nobody knows about it.

Unlike the Oedipus, which articulates desire and law and allows the emergence of otherness, incest erases the limits between family members and introduces a confusion of positions in which nobody knows who is who.

In my opinion, we need to underscore the radical difference between seduction theory, constitutive and foundational of infantile psychosexuality and of repression, which stimulates the representation and constitution of phantasms and leads to the Oedipus complex, on the one hand, and on the other hand, traumatic seduction, and the realm of the deadly. Laplanche (1986) describes the generalized seduction theory by placing the mother in the position as agent of originary or early seduction through the care she gives her baby's body, including breast-feeding and close contact between the mother's body and the child's. This is necessary seduction, Laplanche writes, inscribed in the situation itself.

However, as I stated in a previous paper (Tesone, 1999), the traumatic seduction a child suffers is not part of seduction theory, since sexuality does not operate as a source of life and bonding but, rather, as a persecutory object that unbinds and mortifies. The adult's drive irrupting in the child does not favor the ego's integrity but, instead, leads to the consequence that Green (1993, p. 117) refers to as the "de-objectalizing function of the death drive."

During my 11 years in charge of a center[1] for consultation and ambulatory psychotherapy, specializing in the complexity of problems involved in physical and sexual intrafamilial violence committed against children and adolescents, I interviewed families referred by case workers, following the orders of juvenile court judges. These interviews are not mandatory, but it is obvious that this type of family does not consult unless the

DOI: 10.4324/9781032647791-4

judicial system points out its pathology. The therapeutic team faces the difficult task of eliciting a demand for treatment.

Among the types of intra-familial sexual abuse, I emphasize the most frequent cases: father–daughter incest and the peculiar relation between the incestuous man and his daughter's nascent femininity. Following C. Balier (1996), I insist that it is impossible to understand the perpetrators of incest without first understanding their victims; therefore, it seems appropriate to start with the following disclosure:

Catherine, age 17, was referred to the Center by an educator ordered by the juvenile judge, who suggested that Catherine come to "talk to me about that." To talk about that was to talk about what Catherine had suffered ever since she was 10 years old, regularly, with the apparent banality created by repetition. During the night—but not only nights of the full moon, as in *Kaos*, the Taviani brothers' film—her father abused her sexually, in silence, without exercising explicit physical violence but asking her not to scream: an "extremely delicate" demand to avoid awakening Catherine's older sister, who shared the bedroom. However, her sister had also been abused, according to this father's peculiar idea of paternal equity. Sobbing, hardly daring to look at me, with great modesty, Catherine told me or made me understand that what she most blamed her father for was having deceived her by responding to her immense need for tenderness in a way that was—how to describe it—sensual? erotic? passionate? These words, so easily used when they refer to a love affair, acquire in this case a metallic, cold, hateful connotation. In spite of her current age and womanly body, when Catherine told me this, I heard in her narration the hesitant, choked voice of the little girl she had been the first time: "When I felt the contact of our naked bodies, I told myself, since he's my father, he can't hurt me." And yet...

Her words, once liberated, emerge like stones. But her silence is just as eloquent, or even more so. It is a silence burdened with meaning—or, rather, burdened with lack of meaning, with something unspeakable, unthinkable, and impossible to express, like a hermetically sealed compartment that has cut her off from herself. The incest, barely representable, split off, was kept separate from all narration, from any possibility of communication, with a violence equal to the act she had suffered. Even Catherine's eyes were full of this violence, aimed, of course, at her father, but equally at any adult who, being an adult, could only be her genitor's accomplice. Catherine's mother had died when Catherine was 12. She was so distraught that she could not work through her mourning, instead finding a melancholic way out of this mourning, made impossible by the trauma suffered. Then it became even more difficult, since her father continued to abuse Catherine sexually, thereby making her doubly orphan: orphaned by her mother's death and orphaned by her father, who erased the symbolic paternal function with the incest.

Consequently, Catherine felt that they had stolen her childhood, but especially her femininity, which, she felt, had been emptied, sucked out during the vampire-like encounters with her father. She also felt drowned by persecutory objects: the paternal imago, in its terrifying aspect, of course, but also the maternal imago, sometimes idealized, sometimes accused of "having known" and not having done anything to protect her; perhaps preferring to close her eyes forever rather than to finally open them.

The child as a part-object, experienced as a pseudopod of the parent's ego, has no contingent value for incestuous genitors; their progeny is only narcissistically necessary to satisfy the demand of a filial bond. This filial stipulation signals the structural difference between the pedophile and the incestuous father or mother.

I do not consider it possible to group incestuous parents in any particular nosography, although, following Balier (1996), we could classify them as perversions in a relation of communicating vessels with psychosis.

Paraphrasing Recamier (1992), we may say that incest is not the Oedipus but the diametric opposite. The severe psychopathological configuration that is the incestuous family supports a massive attack on oedipal triangulation by erasing the angles that designate the positions described by its terms: father, mother, and child.

If we consider, with G. Bataille (1957), that transgression lifts the interdiction but does not suppress it, then incest would not be simply transgression of the prohibition of incest. It is as if the prohibition had no representational value for the abusive parent.

The incestuous act, which denies the existence of lack, prevents the child from constituting his or her own subjectivity, a consequence of denial of the child's otherness.

> *The psychotic mother of an adolescent boy 16 years old, Jérôme, said in her delusion that in her future reincarnations she might become her son's sister, or her son might be her father, or even, depending on successive reincarnations, she might become her son's partner.*

This brief psychotic discourse reveals that the incestuous act seeks not only the interchange of bodies but simultaneously embodies the omnipotent wish to occupy all the positions at the same time: to be father–mother–daughter–son at the same time. The incestuous wish, according to P. Legendre (1985), is a wish to be all-powerful: it desires the impossible. The law of prohibition of incest exists to place a limit on this absolute desire. God and the Sacred Family, states Legendre, know nothing about incest, since God lacks nothing.

In his article on incest in Greek mythology, Jean Rudhart (1981) observes that the Greeks condemned incestuous unions, especially those between forebears and their descendants. Reciprocal duties between parents and their children were considered religious. When certain unions were prohibited, it was because, being sacred, the sacred was added to the sacred, which made them hyper-sacred. It was condemned, since the pretense of a man intending, through transgression of a hyper-sacred act, to acquire the divine condition, would sever his anchorage to the human condition.

Beyond drive

The incestuous family lacks the dimension of otherness, since no limits separate its members. These families function as if the group formed a single body that has several heads, like a Hydra. Its equation would be: $1 + 1 + 1 = 1$ rather than $= 3$.

An incestuous father expressed the fear that his adolescent daughter might be attacked sexually on the street, saying, "If something happened to me her. ...." This slip of the tongue reveals the lack of differentiation that ruled this relationship.

The incestuous act negates incompleteness. It is a desperate attempt to avoid confronting, as all human beings must, ambivalence and object loss. Incest seeks to eliminate conflict; it attempts to erase the conflict with the ego that assumes the existence of an irreducible other. With respect to the lack that every human being must confront and is never lacking, the abusive parent functions as if the lack were not fundamental.

The incestuous man does not seek to integrate his inevitably conflictive psychic bisexuality; on the contrary, he would like sexuality and sexual differentiation to be free of conflict.

In these cases, we are far from Freud's conception, which seems to include four persons in every sexual act (letter from Freud to Fliess, 1 August 1899; in Masson, 1985) and alludes to psychic bisexuality. In the case of incest, we cannot even speak of the involvement of two persons, given that the other does not exist.

If we accept the idea as proposed by Lacan (1972, p. 69) that "the woman, not being all, there is (therefore) no sexual relation," we could say that the incestuous man seeks a "complementary" sexual relation, since, in search of completeness, he wants the entire woman to be in him.

In other words, the incestuous father would like to seize femininity through the incestuous act, to appropriate it, at the service of disavowing the difference between the sexes and the generations (Tesone, 1998).

This means that the incestuous father seeks completeness because he is afraid that any narcissistic rending apart might provoke his collapse. He also fears that his daughter's sexuality may revive his infantile sexuality, with its concomitant traumatic effect, the daughter consequently being experienced as the magnifying mirror of the father's pregenital sexuality in its nonintegrated feminine dimension.

In his attempt to achieve his aim, he does not hesitate to demolish his daughter's desire and thereby also her thinking, leaving her psychically destructured— the inevitable result of cumulative traumata that she has suffered.

Through a kind of hypnosis, these children are compelled into a paradoxical immobilization: their silence perhaps reflects the representational vacuum into which they are sucked. The incestuous parent's narcissistic ego envelops the other, conceived as only an extension. The desire of the one is not compatible with the desire of the other. In their "totalizing utopia," incestuous parents experience themselves as the owners of time and death.

Desiring to trap the child in their nets, they propose to ignore that the other, whether phantasm or real, essentially enters a conflictive relation with the ego. The ego of the incestuous parent aims to ensnare the other in its net, but in doing so, the other is devitalized.

Narcissism, writes Green (1983), maintains the illusion of the a-Oedipus (not the anti-Oedipus but the non-Oedipus), since it knows only its own ego. "Like God, the ego considers itself self-engendered and sexless, meaning without sexual limitation and without filiation and therefore with no kinship structure" (p. 73).

The incestuous sexual "relation" can only be an equivalent of masturbation, since the sexuality remains auto-erotic: it is as if the other did not exist. The child's function is reduced to satisfying this object auto-erotism.

The little girl narcissistically seduced by her father dissolves into her father's body. The myth of the One—that is to say, the illusion of being an all-powerful, faultless being—is the phantasm common to abusive fathers. Their children exist only within this ego that considers itself grandiose. The value of the boy or girl is only as a narcissistic appendage.

The abusive parent's attempt could be represented graphically by an open-angled triangle inside a circumscribed circumference. In his expansionistic utopia, the abusive father proposes to erase the angles of the triangle, encompassing it within his megalomania of the One. Since the other disappears, no relation between a self and an other can exist between the abusive father and his daughter; only between himself and himself.

Instead of supporting the exogamous law, the abusive adult intends to be the lawmaker: the maker of a negative, endogamous law in which he appears as an all-powerful, perfect being, the owner of everything. He denies all internal conflict, annexing the other to his narcissism. He seeks double immunity: from his internal conflicts and from the object. He establishes something like an ontological preventive denial of the other's existence. Psychotic repudiation or perverse disavowal are often involved, the other acquiring value as an inanimate fetishistic object.

In these cases, the destructive drives seem to play the role of a last resort in the effort to neutralize the object; they consequently envelop its surrounding reality in the same devastation.

Children who have suffered incestuous relations often have accidents or even directly attempt suicide, expressions of a need for internal punishment. In *Principles of Relaxation and Neo-catharsis*, Ferenczi (1930, p. 93) notes that "parents and adults may go very far in their erotic passion for children," and suggests, as a hypothesis explaining the amnesia following this type of trauma, a "transitory psychosis" that occurs as an initial reaction to the shock. He considers it "a rupture from reality, on the one hand, in the form of a negative hallucination, and, on the other hand, in the form of an immediate positive hallucinatory compensation that provides an illusion of pleasure." This generates "psychotic splitting of a part of the personality that remains secret," which induces psychic self-destruction that paradoxically attempts to protect the psyche from the emergence of anxiety by condemning it to mute suffering.

Quantitative effraction into drive perception induces qualitative damage that is even more devastating when the incest has been repeated over time: acting due to accumulative traumata that impregnate the psyche with death drive.

A triple traumatic effect results: (1) the traumatic quality of the incest itself; (2) the perceptual invalidation often associated with it, in which the adult tells the child that the incest is not incest, thereby denying the gravity of the act; (3) in the incestuous act itself, the child becomes an orphan, since the father and/or mother are still the child's biological parents, but they have erased the symbolic paternal and/or maternal function.

The drama of the incestuous man is that the conflict between the masculine and the feminine is an intra-psychic conflict. This ongoing conflict is acted out in the relationship that is a non-relationship with his daughter, in a desperate body to body struggle to possess the attributes of both a man and a woman: a search for completeness.

Dominant affects in the incestuous relation

Incest does not occur without violence. This violence, sometimes physical but always psychic, develops in an atmosphere that coerces the child.

What do I consider the dominant affect in the incestuous relation? In my opinion, it is hating, based on the death drive that impregnates this link, which is, in reality, a non-link. It could be described as an archaic type of link in which "pregenital love," due to its destructive effects, is not differentiated from hate (Tesone, 2005, p. 54).

In Plato's *Banquet* (c. 385 BCE), Aristophanes' speech discusses the power of love. This text proposes the existence, in ancient times, of three genders: the male, the female, and the androgyne. The latter encompassed the characteristics of the two other genders. It was circular in form as well as in movement. Possessing immense power and pride, it defied the gods. To defend himself from the insolence of the androgynes, and to weaken them without killing them, Zeus cut them in two: "when he had cut one of them, he asked Apollo to turn the head and half of the neck on the cut off side so that the male, seeing the split he had suffered, would be more modest…."

Expelled from the Paradise of plenitude, the man is condemned to separation.

In Aristophanes' myth, each part seeks its complementary half: a fruitless search for lost unity. It is the search for this totality that Aristophanes calls love. Its equation is: $\frac{1}{2} + \frac{1}{2} = 1$. The subject seeks to form an indivisible unit.

In her analysis of the Platonic myths, G. Droz (1992, p. 45) underscores that Socrates expresses himself through Diotima, who considers that love is simply a reunion with the lover's lost part. It renews and fertilizes. It stimulates the beloved, inviting them to create and to be better. It opens the way to something unprecedented: the third party.

In Aristophanes' myth, Droz tells us, love was also tension, but tension directed at the other as a lost part of the self; in the best of cases, the lost fusion was reconstituted.

In contrast, Diotima reasons that love is a dynamic and extroverted tension that stimulates and enriches the other. Its equation would therefore be: $1 + 1 = 3$. Whenever there is an opening for the new, the couple creates something original.

The abusing parent uncloisters himself or herself in the so-called Aristophanist "love" while denying Diotima's description. However, the dominant affect in the incestuous relationship cannot strictly be called love, since destruction of the other always predominates. The incestuous parent does not recoil from his or her search for jouissance: the potential place of anxiety is filled by acting out (Milmaniene, 1995, p. 20). Although this deadly erotization tries to disguise the thanatic dimension, it can only reveal it: "Jouissance, far from the ordering and pacifying shelter of the word and the law, always leads to thanatic positions," according to this author.

The search for absolute jouissance, the attempt to reach the Thing and thereby avoid confrontation with lack, is the impossible aim in incest.

The incestuous act interrupts the chain of generations. It accepts neither progeny nor ancestors; neither origin nor posterity. In Milmaniene's words (2005, p. 29), "only the overcoming of narcissism by recognition of symbolic castration enables the joyful journey from the timeless time of narcissism to the transcendent time of the encounter with the Other." He adds that "the fundamental events forcing the necessary overthrow of narcissism, and the consequent temporalization of time, are therefore: sexuality as recognition of otherness in its irreducible difference, paternity assumed through its gift to the child, and death assumed as creative acceptance of the finite condition." Behind all incest, whatever form it may take, mother–child incest is the same incest Freud brought to light.

There are three versions of the Narcissus myth:

1. In Ovid's version, Narcissus is loved by the nymph Echo. When Narcissus rejects her, she isolates herself so that only her lament is

heard. After a day of hunting, Narcissus goes down to a lake to assuage his thirst, and falls in love with his own image. He does not recognize himself, and when he touches the water, the image disappears.

2. In the Boeotian myth, a young man is in love with Narcissus. Narcissus gives him his sword, with which the youth commits suicide. The scene at the lake is the same as in the first version.

3. In the variation by Pausanias, Narcissus has a twin sister. When she dies, Narcissus suffers unbearable pain. One day, this pain disappears fleetingly when, seeing his image in a lake, Narcissus believes he has seen his sister's image.

Tobie Nathan (1984) interprets the myth of Narcissus, underscoring that, although Narcissus seems to abandon his admirers, it is not really so. Narcissus tends to unite with them, albeit "in a way that confuses subject and object."

The three versions, Nathan says,

> have a common denominator: they evoke, each in a specific register, an attempt to be in one position and simultaneously in the opposite, to be both sender and receiver of his own voice, active and passive, man and woman, and yet himself. When he loves, reunites with, unites with or fuses with his double of the other gender or of the Underworld, Narcissus transgresses a taboo. [p. 15]

F. Héritier-Augé (1944, p. 11) emphasizes that the second type of incest is a crime, sanctioned in certain African communities, since it does not separate what must be kept separate and mixes what should be kept apart, thereby confusing genders, sexes, kinship, and alliance. An accumulation of the identical denies otherness in a mirror search for the double. It is fascination for the identical, the subject's psychic clone and the lethal jouissance of the undifferentiated. The phantasm of the double disavows separation, castration, and death. The double, in the opinion of R. Menahem (1995, p. 119), cannot be considered a return of the repressed but, rather, as the irruption of something unrepresented and unthinkable.

Is the horror of the incestuous act provoked only by transgression of the prohibition of incest, or does it also respond to a transgression of the narcissistic taboo, and thereby multiply its devastating effect?

From the oedipal crossroads to narcissistic mirroring? As J. J. Baranes highlights (1995, p. 39), it seems that Oedipus must often concede his place to Narcissus on our analytic couches, as also occurs in the social and cultural orders. Although the prevalence of Narcissus over Oedipus (Tesone, 2003) characterizes incest, it is perhaps also what generates a difference in contemporary psychoanalytic clinical work, which creates the impression that the incestuous passage to act could be lurking more frequently than in the past. Narcissus lies on our couch more often than Oedipus.

Despotism and sexual abuse[2]

Eurydice, as I will call this patient, did not leave the hell of the prisons of the Argentine dictatorship by the grace of Orpheus, but because of what the military euphemistically termed *"the option."* It meant that, having been considered a political prisoner of the regime and having suffered in prison, neither tried nor sentenced, she was given *"the option"* to go on being a prisoner or to be ostracized, far from her country. Thus, she arrived in Paris, thrust out of a jail in an Argentine province. If you allow me, I would say that, luckily for her, she had been jailed in the months prior to the military coup in March, 1976, so that she was not on the prison records; this allowed her, perhaps, to escape the tragic fate of the "disappeared." She had spent three years, between the ages of 17 and 20, in that jail. Her "crime" had been having pasted up posters against the political regime of the moment, which meant she was considered a "subversive," in the terms of that period. An aid group referred her to me at a hospital service in Paris, where I worked. In this context, we had our first interview. After a short time working face to face, she started an analysis that lasted several years, whose core was the traumatic experiences that marked her life.

In spite of her deplorable physical condition on leaving prison, her graceful feminine traits, nearly adolescent, whose sexual identity had been harshly punished by the prison years, were still perceptible. Practically ever since she had first been imprisoned, anorexia, which exacerbated hair loss, and chronic amenorrhea expressed in her body the intensity of the suffering she had gone through. For obvious questions of limited time, I will not go into the narration of an analysis that extended over several years. From it, I discuss two scenes that are traumatically intertwined.

The conditions in the prison, the overcrowding, the ill-treatment, her disgust at the odor of the latrines permeating the cell she shared with two other female prisoners, were part of the story of the damage suffered. Much later, when her persecutory anxieties and transferential distrust had quieted, she tells me about a scene that was particularly anguishing. She had never told anybody, she explains, maybe not even herself. Stammering, finding it hard to put what had happened into words, she tells me that once, when she was in her cell, an army officer entered. Neither the presence of her cellmates nor her own resistance could prevent the officer from penetrating her vagina with his fingers.

The head of the prison, a higher-ranking officer, found out about it, and could think of nothing better to do—supposedly to determine the facts— than to organize a cross-examination between Eurydice and the violating officer. Face to face with this sinister character, and with the prison chief present, she was unable to make even the slightest accusation: in the first place because, of course, she feared for her life and the violator's reprisals. But in the second place, and she says this between sobs and breathless, because at the moment of penetration she had felt pleasure... And that pleasure, which shamed her, had cancelled out, in her experience, the right to accuse him. She blamed herself; or, rather, she reproached her body, for having betrayed her, for having surrendered to the libidinal violence of the jailer, a detestable person she hated. This experience provoked a feeling of strangeness, almost a psychotic moment of effraction of her personality. This scene, in itself traumatic, later proved to be, not exactly a screen memory, although it did act as a screen, but more precisely what I would call an experience of repetition: in her life, more than once, as she had not been able to use her body according to her own wishes—a body that had been stolen from her repeatedly. From around age 3 until she was 6 or 7, her maternal grandfather had abused her sexually with fellatios and fingering. Since that time, she had been totally unable to get dental treatment, because the many attempts to entrust her mouth to a dentist—that is, to another—threw her into crises of anguish expressed by screaming and crying. Her parents, who had separated, and in particular her mother, with whom she lived, had never expressed the least suspicion of what was going on. Eurydice never could talk about what happened or accuse her grandfather. The repugnance associated with a "strange excitement" made her retrospectively hate her body. At that time, "the option" was also of life or death—not exactly a real death, as in prison, but psychic death. However, in spite of the terror she felt, she was able to break away from these perverse practices to which her maternal grandfather forced her through threats.

This brief double narration of the traumatic shows how the excitement generated in the incested child's body—the effraction of excitement coming in from the outside without consent or desire—produces a traumatic effect. That body, which responds in an uncontrolled way to the external excitation, becomes itself an external body, because of a forcible entry into the ego. This body, which made her feel things, is and is not her body. The excitement produced does not make her desirous, since it is a de-subjectivizing excitation. It is violence added to the violence of the penetration—whether oral, as in her childhood, or vaginal, as in prison. Desire does not intervene; it is a stolen excitement, a swindle, since it sets off drive excitation without the subject's consent. The ultimate trauma is the brutish and brutal encounter with a de-symbolizing event that does not allow the subject to go on ensuring his or her continuity in life (Assoun, 1999, p. 54). The body thus acquires an extraterritorial character, with its own jurisdiction, and requires punishment. It is triply traumatic: because of the effraction and the excessive burden of the fact itself, because of the alienating excitation produced without agreement or desire and because of the experience of de-subjectification it involves. It is jouissance associated with the death drive, a de-fusion of the drives that destructures and annihilates the desiring capacity. The enemy becomes not only the abuser, but also the subject's own body, experienced with shame and even scorn. It is the abused body that "deserves" punishment, because it has forced the subject to feel excitation in spite of herself. A pure, unmet aphorized excitation, pure cathexis mixed with anguish, but excitation at any rate. The damage becomes flesh... in the flesh.

Another female patient, whom I will call Danaid, ate insatiably and mistreated her body with food—a form of oral punishment that the need to flagellate the body may take. As a child, she had suffered incest at her father's hand, in the form of mutual masturbation. Her mother, whom she had tried to tell what was happening, had called her a liar, dismissing her account but, worse yet, even her perception of what had happened. Danaid developed something like a phobia of her own body, which she could hardly bear to see naked in the mirror. Although she was married and had a little girl when she consulted me, it had been nine years since she had had sexual relations with her husband or any other man. Residing in a seaside city, she never went to the beach. She might occasionally go for a walk on the sand, but dressed in long tunics that enveloped her female body, concealed beneath her fat and the clothing she chose to wear. She avoided men's eyes, fearing the slightest possibility of meeting a desiring glance. I would say that Danaid lived painfully with a body that was, supposedly, hers, but which she constantly feared would betray her. Her marriage had become the entrapping situation of infantile impotence, when she could not escape from parental oppression. She had the "advantage" that, unlike what had happened in her childhood, no sexual relationship now awakened feelings in her body. In a paralyzing paradox, by escaping the reign of sexuality experienced traumatically, she also preserved her father as her imaginary partner. Her feelings of shame when others looked at her were humiliating, but that shame allowed her to take a position in relation to her domesticated ideal: the fact that she felt it was proof of her existence as a subject (Assoun, 1999).

When an incestuous father uses his daughter's body to obtain a certain kind of jouissance, he simultaneously denies her condition as a little girl, separate from her father. In a relation that I would define as narcissistic–omnipotent, the father (or sometimes the mother) abuses the little girl or boy in this sense: by denying their status as a subject.

Notes

1 Centre Médico-Psycho-Pédagogique E. Pichon-Rivière, 9 Cours des Petites-Écuries, 75010 Paris.
2 This *section* was previously published as "Stolen Body," in *IDE, Revista de la Sociedad Brasileira de Psicoanálisis*, N° 41, pp. 107–114, Sao Paulo, 2005.

References

Assoun, P.-L. (1999). *Le prejudice et l'idéal. Pour une clinique social du trauma*. Paris: Ed. Anthropos.

Balier, C. (1996). *Psychanalyse des comportements sexules violents*. Paris: PUF.

Baranes, J. J. (1995). *Double narcissique et clivage du moi*. Monographies de la RFP, Le double. Paris: PUF.

Bataille, G. (1957). *L'erotisme*. Paris: Ed de Minuit.

Droz, G. (1992). *Les mythes platoniciens*. Paris: Seuil.

Ferenczi, S. (1930). *Principe de relaxation et néocatharsis* [Principles of relaxation and neo-catharsis]. In: *Psychanalyse, Vol. IV*. Paris: Payot, 1982.

Green, A. (1983). *Narcissisme de vie, narcissisme de mort*. Paris: Éditions de Minuit.

Green, A. (1993). Pulsion de mort. In: *Le travail du négatif*. Paris: Éditions de Minuit.

Héritier-Augé, F.(1994). *Les deux soeurs et leur mère*. Paris: Odile Jacob.

Lacan, J. (1972). *Le séminaire, livre XX, Encore*. Paris: Seuil.

Laplanche, J. (1986). De la théorie de la séduction restreinte à la théorie de la séduction généralisée. *Etudes Freudiennes, 27*: 7–25.

Legendre, P. (1985). *L'Inestimable objet de la transmission*. Paris: Fayard.

Masson, J. M. (Ed.) (1985). *The Complete Letters of Sigmund Freud to Wilhelm Fliess, 1887–1904*. Cambridge, MA: Belknap Press.

Menahem, R.(1995). *Qui a peur de son double?* Monographies de la RFP, Le double. Paris: PUF.

Milmaniene, J. E.(1995). *El goce y la ley*. Buenos Aires: Paidós.

Milmaniene, J. E. (2005). *El tiempo del sujeto*. Buenos Aires: Biblos.

Nathan, T. (1984). La transgression du tabou narcissique. *Cahier U.E.R. Expérimentale de Bobigny, 24*.

Racamier, C. (1992). *Le genie des origins*. Paris: Payot.

Rudhart, J. (1981). De l'inceste dans la mythologie grecque. *Revue Française de Psychanalyse, 45* (4): 732.

Tesone, J. E. (1998). Une activité peu masculine. L'inceste père-fille. *Revue Française de Psychanalyse, 62*.

Tesone, J. E. (1999). De la teoría de la seducción a la seducción traumática teorizada. *Revista de la Asociación Argentina de Psicología y Psicoterapia de Grupo, 22* (2): 198.

Tesone, J. E. (2003). L'incesto e la negazione dell'alterità. *Psicoanalisi: Rivista della Associazione Italiana di Psicoanalisi*: 134.

Tesone, J.-E. (2005). Incest(s) and the negation of otherness. In: G. Ambrosio (Ed.), *On Incest: Psychoanalytic Perspectives*. London: Karnac.

3 From the theory of seduction to traumatic seduction*

When the adult's sexuality breaks into the child's body, breaking down the barrier against para-excitation by effraction, the adult perforates the wrapping that is the child's skin-ego and provokes a traumatic experience whose psychic consequences have serious pathogenic potential. We are quite far removed from the theory of seduction seen as constituting the psychic apparatus. In the case of sexual abuse, I would say that the signifiers are no longer enigmatic, as in the case of original seduction; on the contrary, they are too heavily loaded with signification. This is signification that comes in from the outside and is, for the child, something *too full of significance*, a source of violence. I differ from Laplanche's (1986) conception, in that I consider that the violence lies not so much in the imposition on the child of a need to translate, but in the need, generated in the child, to de-construct that *extra meaning* that doesn't belong entirely to him or her. The enigma is a meaning requiring construction or revelation. *The meaning inoculated into the child by the incestuous parent is a meaning that will have to be de-constructed*. The incestuous parent etches a line on the topology of the child's body surface, drastically modifying the course of his or her libidinal organization and inducing a drive overload that wrenches apart the barrier against para-excitation. The quantitative thus acquires a qualitative value. In "The Aetiology of Hysteria" (1896, p. 209), Freud says in regard to scenes of sexual aggression: "in fact what has taken place is a handing-on, an infection in childhood" by the adult. The image is strong, and it highlights, I think, the idea of invasion, assault, and the permanence of something the abuser has left in the abused beyond the traumatic effect of excessive stimuli. Aside from the purely economic aspect, in function of the drive overload exerted on the child, there is a semantic overload, *an extra significance* that the child must later deconstruct in order to avoid remaining ensnared in the libidinal geography imposed by the aggressor. Although the child is not a *tabula rasa*, on which the incestuous

---

* "De la théorie de la séduction à la séduction traumatique. L'Inceste", presented at the 42nd IPA Congress, Nice, 22–27 July, 2001.

DOI: 10.4324/9781032647791-5

parent writes his or her drives, the course of the child's libidinal organization can be oriented in spite of her or himself. The incestuous act does not libidinize the child's body, as do the parental caresses of primary seduction. Just the opposite: incest freezes or petrifies it and impregnates it with death drive: it is a mark punched in with an awl, which impels the subject to repetition compulsion.

In primary seduction, caresses hold the life drive and tend to fuse the part drives, thus giving the child a chance to try out movements toward integrating a rudimentary body ego.

In traumatic seduction, the death drive predominates, so that instead of encouraging drive integration, it induces a function that Green (1996) terms the de-objectivizing function of the death drive. The child has no status as a subject, but is only a part-object. Sexuality and external–internal are no longer a source of life and fusion, but a deadly persecutory object responsible for the de-fusion of the drives and of thought.

If the death drive is de-objectivizing for the other, it is, at the same time, the same for the subject from which it comes. The more his ego feels threatened by a vacillating and failing narcissism, the more he will want to dominate and subjugate the object, in a desperate attempt to preserve a precarious unity.

At this point, our clinical work puts the following question to psychoanalytic theory: is the object of the drive always contingent? In "Instincts and Their Vicissitudes" (1915), Freud says that "the object is what most variably *is* about an instinct"; he later adds that the object "may be changed any number of times in the course of the vicissitudes which the instinct undergoes during its existence" (p. 123). However, Green (1996) thinks that Freud was not proposing a closed system that would deny the object's importance. In the case of incest in particular, the little boy or girl has no status as a subject, but is a part-object of the part-drives of the abusive parent. In this particular incestuous relationship, I think that the part object–child is not contingent on the abusive father's part-drives. The narcissistic problem so often found in incestuous parents requires the part-object that is closest to hand, in the perspective of narcissistic demand: that is, his own children, as pseudopods, a narcissistic emanation that places them somewhere between a part of his own body and an external object. In these cases, I think that the object of the drive is not contingent, since it demands a filial tie, a displaced path of narcissistic libido. Incestuous parents cannot be classified as pedophilic: they are in a particular category of perversion in which the object of their drives must necessarily have a filial relation with them.

Then, why am I speaking of drives rather than of love or even hate, since these are relationships between parents and their children? It's precisely because I believe that, in this realm of the part drive, we can speak neither of love nor of hate. The child is not a contingent, but rather a necessary object for the abusive parent's fragile narcissistic scaffolding. The incestuous relationship denies the existence of the child separate from the parents. Incestuous parents do not libidinize their children, but vampirize their nascent sexuality, aiming to control in the child what the parents cannot manage to synthesize in their own libidinal organization. This means that their own drive anarchy and the threat it poses to their narcissism are directly proportional to its expansion: the more precarious the narcissistic structure, the greater the expansion. These abusers deny the primacy of everything genital by all means possible, attempting to ignore the castration anxiety that they wish to avoid at all costs. In a previous paper (Tesone, 1998), I proposed the hypothesis that "the incestuous man tries to melt into his daughter's body, to be one with her, stealing her nascent femininity in order to possess the attributes of both sexes". The incested child is a desperate and helpless child in the face of her drives and the external world.

Let us look into the etymological meaning of "seduction," which, in the case of traumatic seduction, acquires its full semantic meaning: from the Latin *seducere*, which means to separate. In traumatic seduction, and even more so in the case of incest, the violence of the intrusion on the child of sexuality loaded with a meaning that does not belong to the child, separates the child from her or himself, from her or his condition as a subject and from a parental function capable of containing the parent's own drives. In order to emerge as a subject of desire, the prerequisite for the child is to *deconstruct the excess significance* and get away from the deadly jouissance that the incestuous parent has inoculated into her developing sexuality, and to be able to recover the symbolic parental function that had been swept away by her own parents through some other adult who is in a position to take it up.

References

Freud, S. (1896). The aetiology of hysteria. In: *Standard Edition, Vol. 3*. London: Hogarth Press, 1962.

Freud, S. (1915). Instincts and their vicissitudes. In: *Standard Edition, Vol. 14*. London: Hogarth Press, 1962.

Green, A. (1996). La sexualité a-t-elle un quelconque rapport avec la psychanalyse? *Revue Française de Psychanalyse, 50* (3).

Laplanche, J. (1986). De la théorie de la séduction restreinte à la théorie de la séduction généralisée. *Etudes Freudiennes, 27*: 7–25.

Tesone, J. E. (1998). Une activité peu masculine. L'inceste père-fille. *Revue Française de Psychanalyse, 62*.

4   *In-cestus*: from disavowal to revelation

Analysis of the film "The Celebration" (*FESTEN*)

The Celebration is a 1998 film of Danish origin. It was the first—and multi-awarded—production of the revolutionary film movement Dogma, a style created by directors Lars Von Trier and Thomas Vinterberg on the basis of a manifesto in which they committed to shoot their films without using music, sets, or artificial lighting, and shooting camera in hand. Trier's ethical proposal is cinema at the service of truth, together with an aesthetic that refuses to put itself at the service of technique and away from the great productions of commercial cinema. The aim of the Dogma collective is to purify cinema by rejecting expensive and spectacular special effects, post-production modifications, and other technical artifices. The filmmakers concentrated on the story and the actors' interpretation. They believed that this approach can most pertinently appeal to the viewer, who is not distracted by overproduction. It is characteristic of this group to film close-ups with a mobile camera, which gives an intimate perspective that highlights, above all, the faces, their expressions, their musings, their furies, their sadness—that is, the emotional aspect of a story where there is no shortage of dialogue, but whose narrative oscillates between the subjectivity denoted by the expression of a face and its group interaction. The collective of the family group is always in filigree, but from the subjectivity of the gaze of each character. All the filming takes place in 24 hours and is made with a video camera. The script takes place in a hotel run by the same family on the occasion of the 60th birthday of the father of the family. It is the occasion to hold a celebration—*Festen,* in Danish—which brings together the closest relatives. From the beginning, we first get to know the adult children of a couple, Helge and Elsie.

A long road through the Danish countryside opens the first scene, in which we see Christian, the eldest son, walking alone along the route. You don't know where the road comes from or where it's going to; it may be a linear path, it may be labyrinth, who knows. We only know that Christian shaved at the airport and that he is "looking at my father's land, which is beautiful," to the point that he wonders if he would want to return. But, like an opera overture that preludes the tragedy that is going to happen, he announces to his telephone interlocutor: "I suppose it will be scandalous."

DOI: 10.4324/9781032647791-6

The tense climate is thus enunciated from the first words, from which the tension continues to rise as encounters and disagreements occur. Michael, the younger brother—an exalted, vociferous character who will reveal himself to be abusive—on seeing his older brother walking along the road, makes his wife and three small children get out of the car, violently, in the name of having the chance of a private chat with his brother, who tries not to accept. The small children, in silence, walking desolate along the route, is the place that the family, we will learn later, reserved for childhood. Other cars arrive; the climate of excitement is mixed with irritability and perplexity. Christian has two restaurants in Paris and Michael a café in a Danish port. Then we meet Helene, an anthropologist sister, with a compulsively addictive relationship with cigarettes. Upon arriving at the family hotel, to Michael's amazement, the concierge announces that he was not on his father's guest list. Filiation falters. His terrible behavior the previous year, due to excessive alcohol, would have meant his exclusion from the party. Once this obstacle has been corrected, the two brothers, their sister, and the other relatives stay at the hotel, reserved entirely for the party. There is talk of a "beautiful funeral," but the viewer does not know from whom, or when it was. The "beautiful funeral" is consistent with an oxymoron, which will not be the only contradiction of the plot. Helene reproaches Michael for not having attended the funeral and not being interested in the family. It is perceived in each of the tense features of their faces, in the movements of their bodies, a barely contained violence, with some equivocal gestures by Michael, such as brushing the breasts of Helene, who warns him without too much conviction that this is not done to a sister. From the beginning, violence—physical or sexual, like the two faces of Janus—will be the true protagonist of the script.

The mother reminds Christian not to forget to congratulate his father on his birthday—a curious request, given that it is the apparent reason for his coming to the family home. He does it formally, dryly, and the father asks him to say a few words for his sister, since he could not do it because he would start crying. His tone, however, is not one of sadness, but hard, imperious, distant. Christian announces that he already has something written. There are scenes in which relatives sing happy birthday to Helge, while he formally embraces his wife. At the same time, in the background, bucolic scenes of park, forest, ducks in a lake, and flowers contrast, in their country-like serenity of pastel colors, with the tensions in the foreground. Although it is not shown, the dialogue suggests another scene, usual for the father as the protagonist and to which the men are invited: the hunt. We will notice later the whole symbolic dimension of this retro scene. Helene is assigned the room where her sister Linda, Christian's twin, had died. The viewer learns that she had committed suicide in the bathroom. They end up finding, with the help of the concierge, a letter from his sister who begins to read but stops, anguished, crying. Due to the intensity of her reaction, it is clear that the content of the letter must be intense, but it is not known what it alludes to. She adds: "No one should find it," as if to avoid its apparent dangerousness.

Various scenes take place in the hotel rooms; their common denominator is sex and violence. Michael beats his wife; the trivial event that triggers it is a pretext, but this extreme violence culminates in a violent sexual relationship between them. A hotel maid, Michèle, Christian's childhood friend, tries to seduce him, but her charm is thwarted by Christian's drug addiction; he faints from an overdose without the relationship having been consummated. The party takes place in a spacious room, elegant, velvety, with sparkling lights that leave no shadows, everything clear and refined. The long dresses of the women and the tuxedos of the men are part of the scenery—scenery that veils the tragedy that is coming. The party takes place in a pre-established order; a guest, Helmuth, is asked to act as occasional master of ceremonies. A smooth character, well kempt, he will do the impossible to avoid tragedy with his relentless sequential order of the party. Its failure will be a success for the truth.

Close-ups of the faces of the protagonists are part of the story, shot with the mobile camera and from a lower plane, highlight the anguished expression of Christian, the dislocated violence of Michael, the alleged bonhomie of the father, Helge, and the stony coldness of Elsie, the mother, whose traditional beautiful features do not hide her sinister look.

They ask Christian to give a speech. He gets up and asks his father to choose which of two texts, one green and one yellow, he prefers. From the smiles of the guests, the night seems playful. The father, perplexed, chooses one text, and Christian reads: "It is the discourse of home truth. I called her when Dad went to the bathroom." The sounds of laughter caused by the announced title do not mask the grimaces. He remembers his twin sister, Linda, "who is already dead," evoking her joy, her smile, and the antics they got up to together as children, which had never been discovered and therefore punished. He continues: "It was more dangerous when Dad took a bath: he would take Linda and me to his study, close the door, lower the blinds, then take off his clothes, undress us… and rape us.… He had sex with his little ones." Facing the astonished look of the guests, he continues: "Two months ago, when my sister died, I realized that Helge [he does not say "dad"] was a very clean man… thanks to so many bathrooms." He continues, lacerated in the tonality of his voice and ironic "and I wanted to share it with the rest of the family, let's celebrate that great person, thank you for all those good years, happy birthday."

The moment of revelation, like a time bomb whose clockwork would have been staged for years waiting to explode, explodes. In the words of Moty Benyakar (Benyakar & Lezica, 2005), the introduction explodes— that is, the foreign body embedded in the psychic apparatus. However, denial, denial does not yet allow the word to reach its symbolic efficacy.

There was a paralyzed silence among the guests. Christian got up from the table and, in private dialogue with the father, apologized, saying he had made a mistake. Helge compels him to leave, wishing him "a good trip," as one might say to a transient client of the hotel. We will never know if the texts were different, but they were probably the same text. Perhaps at last there can be a single, readable text of what really happened, which had, until that moment, been erased from family history. However, struggling inwardly with the father's attempt to expel him and to drown out a truth that has never been revealed, Christian returns to the table, facing the furious gaze of Helge. Paternal grandparents speak, which is not the same as taking the floor: the incoherent, obscene speech of an insane old man with a damaged frontal lobe, whose lack of inhibition represents in the script the lack of inhibitory brakes of the deadly drive of an incestuous father. In aid of Christian's wobbly hesitation, Kim, the hotel's head cook and Christian's childhood friend, plans, with the help of the hotel staff, to support Christian in his complaint. Stealing the keys of the cars so that no one can flee, not only from the hotel, to escape in the face of an uncomfortable situation, but, above all, so that Helge cannot run away from listening and admitting being a violent and incestuous father. Guests are to act in the manner of an oral jury trial that would convict an abusive parent.

In an unexpected plot twist, we see a late guest arrive at the hotel; he is revealed to be Helene's partner. It represents, in the script, the exogamy, the different, which comes from outside to denounce, with its mere presence, the inbred functioning established by these parents. From the logic of his racism, identified with his father's inbreeding, Michael tries to leave him out of the party, denying him his status as guest—something that seems unrepresentable. Helene has to impose, even with physical violence, a man—her partner—in whom everything different: the colour of his skin, the language (he does not speak Danish, but English), his first name, unpronounceable for a Dane: Gbatokai. The scene that follows, during which all the guests sing, in unison, a racist song in Danish, calling Gbatokai a monkey, is one of unusual violence. The arrogance of the homogeneous, vilely questioning the richness of the heterogeneous. Christian takes the floor again, this time to ask for a toast: "For the man who murdered my sister, for the murderer."

The master of ceremonies, in a tragicomic attitude but almost like a Greek choir, asks to be allowed to make an "intermezzo pianissimo," desperately looking for a pause that would allow the denial to be maintained; he orders the pianist to play something "soft"—as if the harmony of music could give melody to the dissonances of an incestuous family. The pretended party begins to fragment, the guests want to leave, violent scenes follow, in particular on the part of Helge towards his son, Christian, whom he accuses of "being sick, of having been an evil child with the other children, of lack of talent with women"; he disqualifies Christian as a person, reducing him to a being without qualities. He accuses him of being a drug addict, of having killed his sister for having migrated and having "abandoned" her. Identified with the mechanisms of negation and denial, as if the script had personified in Helmuth this function of repression and impediment of the return of the cleaved, he tries to resume the "party," or, rather, its simulation. Tears stream down Christian's wiry, livid face. Alcohol flows, seeking to numb intolerable experiences in each of the participants. Elsie comes to her husband's assistance, but is certainly herself, talking, standing, defiantly, and stressing that when Christian was a child, he had a lot of imagination, to the point that he "could not distinguish fiction from reality"; she demands that Christian publicly apologize to his father. Christian, reeling but more forcefully than ever, takes up the floor and denounces the complicity of the mother, accusing her of having been a complacent witness to everything that happened: "I am sorry that you are so hypocritical and corrupt, I wish you death." This is what generates incest, that Thanatos reigns over Eros.

Faced with the collapse of the denial, and in an extreme attempt to silence Christian's truth, Michael and other guests force him out of the room, give him a ferocious beating, they leave him, passed out, in the park—as if secrecy should be guarded, as if truth were more dangerous than denial. We see again how the red thread of the plot is woven of violence, physical and sexual. The master of ceremonies, narrative representative of the denial, tries to continue with the order of the festive tradition and asks Helene to read a letter left by someone in her glass. This is the letter left by Linda, her suicidal sister. Helene, encouraged by her partner, finally begins to read: "Dad has begun to possess me again, although this time it is only in my dreams; I cannot stand it any more, I will leave, as I should always have done." She says goodbye to her beloved brothers, perhaps her only representation of family, without mentioning their parents in the final farewell. Helge, less and less convinced, persists in the denial, praises the letter, and asks for a toast to his daughter Linda. But he can no longer prevent the collapse of the denial: Helge, accompanied by his wife, gets up and leaves. Someone lights a candle, the camera focuses on it occupying the foreground; a faint light is glimpsed and becomes more intense. That play of light and shadow, where the candle flashes, becomes a mutative moment in the film. Christian who has recovered from the beating, after listening to the reading of his sister Linda's letter, faints in the hotel lobby and dreams of her, achieving a posthumous encounter through the dreamlike force of his unconscious. Meanwhile, Michael, drunk, looks for Helge and beats him brutally, to the point that had the guests, called to help by his wife, not stopped him, saving him in extremis, death would have followed. It was Michael's brutish and brutal way, true to form, of removing a father who had actually deprived himself—representative of a primitive talion law, his way of avenging his father's incestuous violence toward his brother and sister.

The guests spend the night at the hotel, and the next morning, breakfast brings them together again. A resurgent and faint hubbub seems to arise. We see relaxed faces, smiles without rictus. Christian, transformed, his look relieved, asks Michèle to live with him. Perhaps only after the revelation, after having suppurated the abscess of trauma entrenched for years, can he think of himself as a desiring subject. The parents approach the table; Helge babbles a speech in which she reluctantly acknowledges the horror of what she committed, and Michael slowly gets up, walks around the table with a weary step, a filmic eternity, until he reaches his father's side, and demands that he now leave. This slow time of the film punctuates the emergence of another time—out of the stagnant time of the traumatic experience, and opening up to the time that flows from life. Helge leaves, embarrassed and self-defeated, but Elsie, his accomplice, remains, defiant, before Christian's puzzled and tormented gaze.

The film masterfully condenses all the incestuous dynamics of a family story over the course of a night, during what was supposed to be a celebration. The viewer discovers that, far from celebrating, from being a celebratory act, the meeting will result in a tragedy the origins of which date back to the childhood of the twins, brother and sister. The times, as the times of the unconscious overlap, the denial and cleavage mechanisms collapse, and only after the revelation of incest can the truth be glimpsed, lacerating, but repairing a scar until that had until that moment, been open. The deadly, incestuous father causes the real death of Linda and the near psychic death of Christian, whose drug addiction never managed to appease his suffering. The technique of moving close-ups gives a particular relief to each subjectivity—Christian's suffering, but also that of Michael, beyond his violence; Helene's, who had for years wanted to move away from an inbred dynamic, desperately seeking exogamy through the exact opposite, but achieving it only partially—to such an extent that, having discovered the accusatory letter of her sister Linda, who committed suicide, she does not manage to spontaneously denounce the father until after a long detour, and thanks to the insistence of Christian. The height of trauma "is that brute and brutal encounter, with a de-symbolizing event that no longer allows the subject to ensure his vital continuity" (Assoun, 1999, p. 54). The body thus acquires a character of extraterritoriality, with its own jurisdiction, which needs to be punished. It is triply traumatic: through the fraction and overload of the fact itself, through the alienating excitement produced without agreement or desire, and through the experience of de-subjectivation that it implies. The body is associated with the death drive, detachment from the drives that deconstruct and annihilate the desiring capacity. The enemy becomes not only the abuser, but also the body itself, lived with shame and even contempt. It is the abused body that "deserves" punishment for having made itself feel, in spite of arousal—an excitement that is not metaphorical, pure charge, mixed with anguish. The damage becomes body... in the body. Linda can't shake off the deadly incest, and her guilt and shame will probably compel her to suicide. Death is the only way out of ignominy. Helge, like many incestuous parents, denies incompleteness, in a desperate attempt to avoid confrontation—to which every human being is subject—with ambivalence and the loss of the object. Incest seeks conflict, trying to erase the conflict with the self that supposes the existence of an irreducible other. If the fault is never lacking, the incestuous father pretends, on the contrary, that there may be no fault. To try to achieve his ends, he does not hesitate to demolish the desire and therefore the thought of the child leaving him in a state of psychic destructuring—the inevitable consequence of the cumulative traumatisms to which he is subjected. The child, through a form of hypnosis, is compelled to paradoxical immobilization; His silence perhaps reflects the representational vacuum into which he has aspired. That silence can last for years, sometimes for almost a lifetime. We don't know Christian's age, but by the time he manages to break his silence, 30 to 35 years have probably passed. The incestuous father's self tries to trap the other in his net, but in doing so devitalizes him. The narcissistic self of the incestuous father encompasses the other conceived as a mere extension of self. The desire of the one is not compatible with the desire of the other. The incestuous family lacks the dimension of otherness, there being no limits that separate them. They are families that function as if the group formed a single body and several heads, like a hydra. His equation would be as follows: 1+1+1=1 and not 3 (Tesone, 2008). In his totalizing utopia, the incestuous father lives as master of time and death. Wanting to include the child in their networks, they try to ignore that by essence the other, whether fantastical or real, enters into a conflictive relationship with the self. In the case of incest, the object is present but does not acquire a status of subject, but that of part-object in the form of a narcissistic appendage. Deadly in its essence, since the incessant contribution of excitement is not elaborated by the child. The myth of the One—that is, the illusion of being an all-powerful and flawless being—is the common ghost of abusive parents. His offspring exist only within that self that pretends to be great. The child has no other value than that of narcissistic appendix. Christian, Linda, Helene, and Michael, denied as subjects, did not acquire filial value for Helge; but not for Elsie, either.

From the moment he used the twins to satisfy his impulses; Helge removed himself from his paternal function and excluded his children from his filiation. It is no coincidence that, in the script, when Christian recites the facts of rape by his "father," he does not speak of "father" but, laconically, of "Helge", that is, a person who has a first name, but whom he does not recognize as his father but as a mere rapist. Transgressing the family prohibition—says Barthes (1971, p 141)—consists of altering the terminological sharpness of parental cutback, making a single meaning (a girl named "Olympia," as in Sade's novel *Justine*) simultaneously be given several names—that is, it has the triple honor of being at the same time my daughter, my granddaughter, and my niece. To transgress is to name outside the division of the lexicon, says Barthes: transgression appears from this perspective, as a surprise of nomination. Barthes points out that

incest consists in transgressing a semantic rule, in creating homonymy—
that is, deep down, incest is a surprise of vocabulary. The adult abuser,
instead of being the support of the exogamous law, pretends to be the
maker of the law, but a negative, inbred law, where he presents himself as
an all-powerful and flawless being to whom everything belongs. It denies
the child his or her status as a subject, separate from his or her father. It
is common to find as a psychic structure narcissistic perversion, in which
perversity aims to deny the existence of the psychic reality of the other,
aims to destroy or reduce it.

Near the end of the film, when Helge finally admits the abuse he has
committed with his children, he spits at Christian a terrible phrase: "you
were only good for that," attributing to him a value of a fetishized part-
object that satisfied his drives, denying him his status as a subject. The
incestuous father denies all internal conflict by attaching the other to his
narcissism with respect to regarding their internal conflicts and regarding
the object. Psychotic foreclosed or perverse denial is often at play, often
taking the value of an inanimate fetishistic object. Thus, the impulses of
destruction seem to play the role of last resort, seeking to neutralize the
object, encompassing the reality that surrounds it in the same devastation. Ferenczi (1932), in his famous article on the confusion of tongues between child and adult, stressed precisely that confusion comes from the
fact that the adult responds to the child's request for tenderness with the
language of eroticization. The child's first reaction, Ferenczi says, would
be rejection, hatred, disgust, violent resistance. However, to the extent that
coercion persists, and by introjection of the aggressor, the latter disappears as an external reality. The aggressor does not feel guilty, because he
projects the guilt on the child. And the child, by introjecting the feeling of
guilt that is evacuated by the adult, then demands punishment. And that
punishment is often exercised on one's own body, which, in a cleavage
of the self, is held responsible for having had experiences of excitement
despite the repugnance of the act. It is common for children who have
lived through incestuous relationships to have eating disorders, repeated
accidents, or even outright suicide attempts, as an expression of a need for
internal punishment, as happened with Linda. Ferenczi (1932) writes that
parents and adults can go very far in their erotic passion for children; he
suggests as a hypothesis that the amnesia that follows this type of trauma
is a temporary psychosis, the first reaction to shock. He conceives it as a
break with reality, on the one hand, in the form of negative hallucination,
and on the other in the form of immediate positive hallucinatory compensation that gives an illusion of pleasure. A psychotic cleavage of a part of
the personality that remains secret is generated, inducing a psychic self-
destruction, which paradoxically seeks to protect it from the emergence of
anguish and condemns it to mute suffering. If Linda, through her suicide,
was mute forever (although her letter also had a belated word effect), luckily for Christian the traumatic experience did not leave him totally mute,

and, as is common in this type of trauma, he could finally speak, after many years had elapsed. Linda's death perhaps gave him strength to shed the deadly family "secret." The fraction of the quantitative, of the perceptual impulsion, induces an even more devastating qualitative damage to the extent that incest has been repetitive over time; acting by cumulative trauma, which permeates the psyche of death drive.

There is a triple traumatic effect: (1) the traumatic excess of the burden; (2) often associated perceptual disqualification (the adult tells the child that incest is not incest, i.e., denies the seriousness of act): (3) in the very act of incest, the child becomes an orphan (the father and/or mother remain the biological parents but have erased the paternal and/or maternal symbolic function). The traumatic effect can be visibly immediate or become entrenched and act much later, as a real time bomb. When the sexuality of the adult makes irruption in the body of the child by breaking the barrier of para-excitement, the adult pierces the envelope represented by the skin ego of the child and causes a traumatic experience, with psychic consequences that have a serious pathogenic potentiality.

The incestuous parent inscribes a trace in the topology of the child's body surface, dramatically modifying the course of his libidinal organization and inducing a drive overload that tears the para-arousal barrier. Although the child is not a *tabula rasa*, in which the incestuous father imprints his drives, the course of the child's libidinal organization can be oriented in spite of himself. The incestuous act does not libidinize the child's body, as do the parental caresses of primary seduction. On the contrary, incest freezes the child, petrifies him, and impregnates him with the death drive, a mark traced with an awl that impels him to compulsion to repetition. In traumatic seduction, the death drive predominates, which, instead of favoring impulsive integration, induces a function that Green (1993) calls "the de-objectifying function of the death drive." The child does not have a status of subject, but of part-object. Sexuality, external–internal, no longer becomes a source of life and bonding, but a deadly persecutory object responsible for the unmixing of impulses and thought. If the death drive is de-objectifying for the other, it is also simultaneously de-objectifying for the subject from whom it emanates. The more he will feel his ego threatened by a vacillating and faltering narcissism, the more he will want to dominate and tame the object in a desperate attempt to preserve a precarious unity. And in that struggle, Helge obtains the complicit connivance of his wife. Incest, beyond the fact that the passage to the act may be individual, is often the effector of an incestuous parental relationship, in which both parents have a shared responsibility, in a kind of *"folie à deux."* Incest is not inscribed in the linear continuation of the Oedipus complex. On the contrary, in the serious incestuous family psychopathological configuration, there is a massive attack on Oedipal triangulation, with erasure of the vertices that designate the places described by the functions of father, mother, and child. Incest is not Oedipus, but the diametric opposite. The abusive parent's attempt could be plotted as a triangle whose vertices do not close, included in a circumscribed circumference. In his expansionist utopia, the abusive father seeks to erase the vertices of the triangle, encompassing it in his megalomania of the One. Between the abusive parent and the child, there is not a relationship of self to an other (disappearing), but one of self to self (Tesone, 1998).

Contrary to Oedipus, which articulates desire to symbolic law, allowing the emergence of otherness, incest erases the boundaries between family members and introduces confusion between them—confusion of places (it is no longer known who is father, mother, son, daughter) and therefore confusion between generations. Eros puts himself at the service of Thanatos and makes traumatic effraction in the psychic life of the instated child, generating a state of destructuring shock and therefore annihilating his psychic life. Incestuous intercourse is frozen in a certain kind of object autoeroticism: the child's body is experienced by the incestuous father as part of his own body in an omnipotent narcissistic attitude. The child expects affection and tenderness from his parents, and the tragic confusion is installed when the father or mother responds with the language of eroticism, imposing an apparent trivialization, almost as a style of communication that sometimes lasts years, where the whole family knows and denies at the same time. As emphasized by the Ortigues (1966), no one can say who is who without making a certain number of choices between the logical possibilities offered by language that allude to place value: one is son or daughter, father or mother, brother or sister, and so on. The prohibition of incest holds a logical function without which everything would be obscured by confusing the boundaries of each. The important thing about the possibility offered by parenthood is not the place of biological genitor, but the ability to exercise the maternal and/or paternal symbolic function. For the child to emerge as a subject, a family symbolic order is required. This order presupposes the existence of differences between generations as well as the distinction between the sexes, so that the *princeps* function of the family, whether traditional or assembled, which is to produce alterity, can be effective symbolically. It's what Helge and Elsie have blocked in their children, unleashing violence and death between them and that the Dogma movement condensed into a masterful *mise-en-scène*, where the scenes multiply and clarify each other, both with their narrative in images and with the narrative of close-ups filmed with a mobile camera. There are no shots that seek effectiveness, the scenes of sexual abuse and incest are narrated by Christian, and read from a posthumous letter left by Linda, Christian's twin sister who committed suicide. There is an intertwining between the images and the discourse that enhances the outcome of the tragedy. The image acquires a subjective value through the close-ups of faces that speak, with words and gestures. It is very suggestive to conclude provisionally regarding the bond that unites verb and image—that is, what cinema can contribute to the discourse in psychoanalysis, as proposed by Jacques Ancet (2013) in one of his poems:

On voit, oui. Mais quoi?	One sees, yes. But what?
Ce qu'on entend.	What he hears.
Comment ça?	How can this be?
Des images dans l'oreille.	Images in the ear.
Dans l'oreille?	In the ear?
Oui, là où parle la voix.	Yes, where the voice speaks.
Et que dit-elle?	And what does it say?
Ce qu'onvoit.	What you see.

References

Ancet, J. (2013). *Portrait d'uneombre & Retrato de una sombra* [Bilingual edition], trans. C. Madero. Buenos Aires: Alción.

Assoun, P.-L. (1999). *Le préjudice et l'idéal. Pour une clinique social du trauma*. París: Ed Anthropos.

Barthes, R. (1971). *Sade, Fourier, Loyola*. París: Seuil.

Benyakar, M., & Lezica, A. (2005). *El proceso traumático*. Buenos Aires: Biblos.

Ferenczi, S. (1932). Confusion of tongues between adults and the child. *International Journal of Psychoanalysis, 30* (No. 4, 1949): 225–230.

Green, A. (1993). Pulsión de mort, narcissisme négatif, fonction désobjetalisante. In: *Le travail du négatif*. Paris: Ed. de Minuit.

Ortigues, M. C., & Ortigues, E. (1966). *L'oedipe africain*. Paris: Plon.

Tesone, J. E. (1998). Une activité peu masculine. L'inceste père-fille. *Revue Française de Psychanalyse, 62*.

Tesone, J. E. (2008). Los incestos y la transgresión del tabú narcisista. In: *Los laberintos de la violencia*. Buenos Aires: Ed. Lugar & the APA.

5 Dominique

Incest in the folds of the name or *ig-nominia**

There was a phone call to my office at the time of my life when I was residing in Paris. I heard a woman's voice, and the distance between the ease of expressing herself and the tone of a little girl surprised me. During the interview that followed her request, I received a woman in her forties (I will call her Dominique). She was very elegantly dressed, in clothes that wrapped her completely. A brilliant lawyer, her professional life was crowned with success. Her emotional life was still intense, although Dominique never shared her daily life with a partner, preferring to create relationships in which she retained a mastery of distance. Battling a depression that could compromise her professional activity, she chose to come and see me, knowing that, at the time, I was responsible for a psychotherapy center[1] that specialized in problems of physical and sexual violence. I later understood that her consultation was guided by the idea that my institutional function would allow me to be closer to a hitherto unspoken story. Having heard in this context unspeakable accounts of incest, her own account "would not leave her out of the human condition."

When she was 12, Dominique had been deflowered by her father. On the basis of his condition as a clinician, the incestuous act was perpetrated on a stretcher in his office; the penetration was carried out digitally, in the name of medicine and the supposed necessary knowledge that a doctor must have about the body of his patient, even his daughter. This scene was repeated for years, until Dominique felt compelled to leave the family home at 18, the only possible form of psychic survival.

Her father, highly respected in his professional environment, occupied a place of unquestionable power among his colleagues and in his family. Every time this doctor by vocation approached his daughter's body, Dominique felt, while her father ran his hands over her body, that he intended to appropriate it, empty it of its contents, make it his own,

* First published as: "About the lie in its protective function of psychism. Dominique: incest in the folds of the name or *ig-nominia*." *Revista de Psicoanálisis*, Vol. 72, No. 4, Asociación Psicoanalítica Argentina, Buenos Aires, 2015.

DOI: 10.4324/9781032647791-7

vampirize her nascent femininity—as if demanding of her that she make him an immobile offering, in the name of a pretended filial love frozen in a deadly scenario. Dominique's father could have violent crises of rage at the slightest movement of autonomy on her part, so that she had been unable to practically create friendships with girls or boys of her age. The rare times Dominique tried to rely on her mother to warn her of what was happening, she only found a wall with no ability to listen in her passive collusion. The same happened with one of her sisters, the other person in her family who had also been encouraged to speak. Without finding a reaction commensurate with the gravity of the story, she was abandoned to her helplessness. In the development of the cure, I understood that my work in the area and the significant number of stories of incest that I had been able to hear made me, in her imagination, an interlocutor capable of understanding her. Her expectation was that my listening would allow her to get out of the traumatic cystic confinement whose impassable wrapping confined her to a desperate solitude. At the same time, sifted through my institutional experience, my condition as a psychoanalyst, necessary for listening to her, was not going to prevent me from taking into account the factual nature of her perception in the chain of her traumatic experience.

It often happens that, in this type of psychic damage suffered repetitively, to the traumatogenic effect of incest itself, the perceptual disqualification is added to the traumatogenic effect of incest. The abusive father commits the incestuous act and at the same time tells the girl that it is not incest, as if it were an act of love and not deadly, an enunciation that oscillates between negation and denial. This perceptual disqualification is doubly maddening since it attacks the perception of the girl, leaving her in a state of psychic collapse due to not being able to trust her own perceptions, and in a state of orphanhood for the loss of the father, since in the incestuous act there is murder of the paternal function. "Death of the soul," Schreber would say (Freud, 1911). Only one blurred genitor remains. The nascent femininity vampirized, her perceptions disqualified, her thinking attacked, Dominique remained mute for 22 years before she could "tell" it to someone outside her family environment. She chose a therapeutic framework. Belonging to an inbred medical family herself, my own medical training was distressing to her, but my condition as a foreigner in France, conversely, relieved her. It offered her a possible exogamous experience.

After about six months of analysis, one day, evoking in session the children that her father had had from a second marriage, Dominique tells me of the disgust she felt every time her father, apparently committing a lapse, addressed her half-sister with her own name, calling her Dominique, as if confusing her with her. I tell Dominique that she probably experienced it as if her father, in pronouncing her name, seized her half-sister's body, as if he possessed her, as if he appropriated her body, as he had done to her. It was then, and only then, that Dominique told me that the first name and surname with which she presented herself to the consultation were not real: she had come up with aliases. Only after my intervention did I understand why I had had this need for masking. That is to say, for months she presented herself to me with a "false" identity. Since being a psychoanalyst is not equal to the profession of notary and even less of police, with no patient would I think of demanding an identity document. After all, it is a matter during a cure of accessing the subjectivity of the patien, which we do not confuse with the social identity she chooses. In a previous work (Tesone, 2011), I had the opportunity to describe how the first name comes to indelibly seal the body of the child, giving him or her the right to be recognized in his or her unique identity. The name, like the skin, contains the child, marks the boundary between their body and the body of the other. Hiding their name, cross-dressing it, dressing in wraparound clothes, was Dominique's way of protecting her body from domination by the other, as a last barrier around her skin ego, as a wall behind which her femininity would have been protected from all incestuous vampirization. Her paranoid transference anxieties, prevalent at the beginning of the cure, were transformed, thanks to the confidence acquired in a progressively positive transference. Dominique finally gave me her real first name—a detail with its own importance, as her real name was bisexual (indeed, like Dominique, the fantasy name chosen to present this patient, in French some names are written or pronounced in the same way, either for women or for men, without marking gender difference). Curiously or not, Dominique's name was the same as her father's, a ghost of hermaphroditism so common with incestuous parents, and sealed in the case of Dominique and her father by the consubstantiation of their two identical names. The last name, which I never got to ask her, she would tell me spontaneously only after a year of treatment. The field of the traumatic interrogates in a paradigmatic way the unrepresentable, putting in tension the classic analytic device of making the unconscious conscious and revealing that in this clinic the lifting of repression is not enough for the trace of something anemic to become mnemic. It is well known that traumata are disruptive experiences, as suggested by Moty Benyakar (2006), that having failed the linking between psychic representation and affect representation could not be represented. Outside the figural, the representable, the traumatic experience escapes the domain of the symbolic and therefore remains suspended in a fixed, stopped, unworkable time. Benyakar (2006) affirms that the essence of the traumatic is the irruption in the psyche of the heterogeneous, the non-own, without the possibility of metabolizing it by transforming it into one's own. What is the status of that which has been lived without being experienced?—something that is part of the psyche without being represented, and not having been symbolized, has not been able to be subjectived? The subjects who have suffered a disruptive experience that turned traumatic worry because they remain in a no man's land on the border. A-structured rather than structured, but not unstructured, they do not decide to belong to any classical nosography; they do not have those letters of nobility. Or, rather, the letter is not written with an accurate pen. In the words of several girls who had suffered incest and were in psychotherapy in a center that specialized in this problem, for which I had responsibility for several years, the disruptive appears (Tesone, 2005), in filigree, through the story of the excitement that had been generated in the girl's body by the physical stimulation coming from outside, without agreement or desire. Such a body, which responds uncontrollably to external excitement, becomes itself an external body, in an unfolding of the self. That body that made her feel things is and is not her body. It is a body that it does not recognize as its own. The excitation produced does not, however, make it desirous, since it is a subjective excitation. It is a violence added to the violence of penetration. Desire does not intervene, it is a stolen excitement, and it is a scam, since it triggers the impulsive excitement without the consent of the subject. The height of trauma is that brutish and brutal encounter with a de-symbolizing event that does not allow the subject to ensure his vital continuity (Assoun, 1999). The body thus acquires a character of extraterritoriality, with its own jurisdiction, which needs to be punished. It is triply disruptive: by the fraction and overload of the fact itself, by the alienating excitement produced without agreement or desire, and by the experience of de-subjectivation that it implies. It is a joy associated with the death drive, detachment from the drives that deconstructs and annihilates the desiring capacity. The enemy becomes not only the abuser, but also the body itself lived with shame and even contempt. It is the abused body that "deserves" punishment for having made you feel excitement in spite of itself, in a sinister unfolding of the Self. As if the girl said, "It didn't happen to me, it happened to my body.... It wasn't me"—an excitement not metaphorical, pure charge, mixed with anguish, but excitement at last. The damage becomes body... in the body. The girl thus feels disqualified as a subject, subject to an experience not experienced as her own. In my opinion, in this clinic, the work of the analyst is not only to lift repression to favor remembrance. As Viderman (1970) suggests, in this case, the analyst's job is not to unveil a hidden sense, but to construct a sense that had never been formed before the analytic relation. According to Green (1990), the analyst forms an absent sense. It creates the necessary conditions so that the potentially traumatic disruptive experience can be qualified, thought, lived, said, more here than the historical truth, but close to the experiential truth in its perceptual qualification. The discourse of trauma, says Françoise Davoine (1998), is always carried by someone de-subjectivated from the knowledge inscribed in the body, to such an extent that it suspends both the judgment of attribution and the judgment of existence. If time is stopped, it is because for there to be time, it is necessary that there be subject, and for there to be subject and therefore repression, a succession of signifiers is necessary. In the case of trauma, the chain of signifiers is interrupted, and that is precisely where time stops, waiting for a new signifier. The usual regression in the cure would lead us not so much to a remembrance, as is usual in the analysis of neurotics, but to an area of representative ambiguity in which the representation becomes diffuse, lost in a cone of shadow. To find it, or even to produce it, would be the crossroads. But this construction requires a previous step, which is the deconstruction of what officiated as defense—that is, the cyst of non-representation that remained cleaved as a pure mark waiting for meaning. The construction achieves, in the best of cases, that the membrane of the cyst becomes porous and the representative-affection of the drive crosses the barrier entering to circulate, fluidly and without reluctance, through the chain of unconscious signifiers. The hole in the chain of signifiers will no longer be a void that aspires towards nothingness of all meaning, but from the new sense will act as an engine of construction of meaning. In patients subjected to disruptive experiences that have become traumatic, the narrative Self is emptied of substance, an impersonal voice coming from afar, from I do not know what memory or what forgetfulness. We don't know who speaks and to whom he speaks. Does the other speak in me? Does the voice speak of the cyst that replaced it? The person performs an endless search for an I, which, while always in its essence dehiscent and unfinished, can nevertheless achieve harmony with the subject. In order to gain access to their own Self, connected from their conscious and unconscious affections, the narrative must be decanted from a flow of words lost in the haze of emotional–perceptual ambiguity, which, beyond their associative value, fail to convey the emotions folded into the defensive cyst. More than a monolithic and immovable tower, the instance of the Self is like a figure of variable geometry in continuous transformation, which, despite its polyhedral character with multiple facets that refract its fragmentary character, does not define the subject, but places it at the axis of its emotional responsibility. The analyst, a historian who seeks to restore not the historical truth of the facts, but the experiential truth of the subject, cannot completely abandon this search either. Although it is known that the search for historical truth is destined to fail, neither can the intervention of the analyst be based on a construction that is totally independent of the perceptual of the truth of the facts. It is perhaps necessary to maintain a permanent tension between the search for historical truth and mythical construction, so that it does not run the risk of becoming a meticulously constructed but wobbly delirium, to such an extent that the subject does not stand up. Otherwise, there is a risk that the analytic process acquires a strong load of projective suggestion on the part of the analyst. Contrary to social discourse, what is said in a cure is not opposed to the unsaid. It is convenient, however, to differentiate between the enigmatic, the domain of the unconscious, of the lie (associated with the secret), and the domain, in part, of consciousness.

The *"tell me everything that goes through your head without reluctance or value judgment"* is the classic slogan of a cure with which we torment the patient, a persecutory paradox slip, since the unsaid or even the lie may have, at least temporarily, a beneficial quality for the discourse of the analytic session. Resource of independence with respect to resistance and defense mechanisms allows the acceptance of the weight of the signifier and the time of meditation and understanding necessary for the elaboration. Lying assumes that you know what you are lying. However, lying covers a vaster semantic field, which includes ignorance of everything that is lied to or the function it fulfills. In the evolution of the child's psyche, lying gives them the opportunity to escape parental omnipotence, assuring them the possibility of building their own independent inner space. Piera Castoriadis-Aulagnier (1976) argues that the discovery that speech can tell the truth or a lie is as essential for the child as the discovery of sex difference, mortality, or the limits of the power of desire. In Dominique's case, making her real name known put her at risk of incest and of exposing her body to the domination of the other, as she had suffered in her childhood. The lie served a function of protecting her narcissistic armor. In that sense we could say that the lie operated as the reserve of a reluctant signifier, since it is never the gross product of a reality, however traumatic it may be, and that it requires time of elaboration to draw its veil. Pretending to extract the secret of the other, denouncing the lie is an inquisitorial process that is far from the psychoanalytic method. It would be to leave it empty, to demolish its resistance, to annihilate it. It would have been useless to rush to know the social identity of Dominique through a long-silenced surname after she entrusted me with her first name. One can evoke the failure of the father's name, a faint symbolic operation in the case of incest, but not to be confused with the surname. I believe that Dominique's lie regarding their names had the function of invoking a name that, although fictional, was the bearer of symbolic castration and acceptance of the fault, underpinning its fragile narcissistic scaffolding. In the change of their names, she moved away from paternal domination, able to paradoxically be herself in the axis of her untainted subjectivity. If the lie was held so firmly, it is because it constituted the key that opened the chain of signifiers and allowed it, at the same time, to remain protected from premature triggering. It was through incest that Dominique became an infringement in her subjectivity, but, paradoxically, it was through lying that she was able to preserve her identity from the fear of effraction, avoiding the risk of repetitive harm. She kept the lie until the transferential moment was propitious for her to leave the incestuous cavern and open herself to a light that would not blind her. The coming to the light from the shadows of the cave of the Platonic allegory is not simple; and, on the other hand, it does not bring good luck to identify massively with the fate of Oedipus in tragedy, famously blinded. Incest leads to tragedy. The Oedipus complex, on the other hand, understood symbolically, allows the assumption of lack and symbolic castration: it is the computer of subjectivity, it is an Oedipus without tragedy, structuring. In the framework of a cure, the subject has the freedom to tell the truth or to lie: the important thing is not to elucidate it hastily but to lead the patient to think the forbidden, to think the unthinkable, and work through her unconscious truth. The provisional lie may have a function that perhaps prevents you from wanting and thinking in your own name.

Note

1 Centre Médico-psycho-pédagogique E. Pichon-Rivière, 9 Cour des Petites, Écuries, 75010 Paris.

References

Assoun, P.-L. (1999). *Le préjudice et l'idéal. Pour une clinique sociale du trauma*. Paris: Anthropos.

Benyakar, M. (2006). *Lo disruptivo*. Buenos Aires: Biblos.

Castoriadis-Aulagnier, P. (1976). Le droit au secret. Condition pour pouvoir penser. *Nouvelle Revue de Psychanalyse, 14*: 141–158.

Davoine, F. (1998). *El discurso analítico del trauma*. Seminar transcribed from recording, given at the Ministry of Health, Department of Mental Health, Province of Buenos Aires, Argentina

Freud, S. (1911). Psycho-analytic notes on an autobiographical account of a case of paranoia. In: *Standard Edition, Vol. 12*. London: Hogarth Press, 1958.

Green, A. (1990). *La folie privée*. Paris: Gallimard.

Tesone, J.-E. (2005). Incesto. El cuerpo robado. *Revista IDE. Sociedad Brasileira de Psicoanálisis de San Pablo, 41*: 107–114.

Tesone, J.-E. (2011). *In the Traces of Our Name*. London: Karnac.

Viderman, S. (1970). *La construction de l'espace analytique*. Paris: Denoël.

6   A pain without a subject[*]

The concept of fantasy in Freud inevitably refers to the concept of perception, based on what is inscribed in the subject from conscious or unconscious perceptions. Now, if Freud considers that in fantasy construction, as in dreams, the subject is always present, could we say that a person may have sensory experiences, events that remain outside the subjective field and, therefore, of fantasy? Furthermore, if this were true, what meta-psychological status and implications would they have in clinical work with whatever provokes a lasting psychic effect, an effect of memory outside the field of the lifting of repression and of fantasy? Is there parental lack that could produce psychic inscription without a subject (Tesone, 2009)?

Psychoanalysis in the past twenty years has turned its interest not only towards fantasy, but also to what may be figured or represented, in opposition not so much to what may not be represented as to what is not represented, but rather inscribed. As highlighted by Sara and Cesar Botella (1992), non-representation originates neither in repression nor in denial and is not an effect of the castration complex or the product of an ego mechanism. It is by taking into consideration a hole, a negativity manifested in psychic dynamics in the form of an alteration of a process, most frequently expressed as a defect in thinking, that they postulate it as being like a memory without memories. In this regard, we re-encounter Bion's (1962) proposals regarding thoughts without a thinker.

The field of the traumatic paradigmatically questions what cannot be represented, putting the classical analytic device of making conscious the unconscious in tension and revealing that in this clinical work, it is not enough to lift repression in order to enable a somewhat anaemic trace to become memory. Traumatic experience sometimes generates emptiness of figuration that swallows up any possible form of representation, prior to fantasy. How does inscription acquire perception of the disruptive fact?

[*] First published in *Changing Sexualities and Parental Functions in the Twenty-First Century*. London: Karnac, 2017.

DOI: 10.4324/9781032647791-8

My objective is to open a road rather than to indicate an itinerary with respect to this enquiry. "Her childhood had injured her to such a degree that she could not evoke it", suggests Quignard (1998, p. 35, translated for this edition), referring to Nemie, the protagonist of his novel, *Vie Secrète* [Secret Life]. I would add, perhaps because pain might sweep away the possibility to represent it, too; non-figuration is a defence against unspeakable pain. "What pain are you talking about if I didn't feel it…" could be the eloquent phrasing of this extreme psychic resource. Duras (1964, p. 47) writes of Lol V. Stein in her novel, *Le Ravissement de Lol V. Stein*, "suffering had not found in her anywhere to slip out". Later in the same novel (p. 58, translated for this edition) she wonders, "But what does suffer without a subject mean?"

In his paper, "Fear of Breakdown", Winnicott (1974) states that this is perhaps fear of a past event whose experience has not yet been undergone. The need to go through this experience is equivalent to what, in the analysis of neurotics, might be the need to remember.

As we know, experiences are traumatic when they are disruptive, as Benyakar (2006) suggests, having caused processes of binding to fail, rendering them incapable of representation. Outside of what may be figured or represented, traumatic experience escapes the domain of the symbolic and, therefore, remains suspended in a fixed, slowed-down time that cannot be worked through. Benyakar (2006) states that the essence of the traumatic is invasion of the psyche by something heterogeneous, extraneous, impossible to metabolize, and which, thereby, transforms into something of one's own.

What is the status of something that has been experienced without being experienced, which is part of the psyche without being represented, that, not having been symbolized, has not been able to be subjectivized? In any case, we are far from fantasy and the intrinsic inclusion of the subject in the scene to which Freud referred. Subjects who have suffered disruptive experience that has become traumatic are disquieting because they remain in a "no-man's-land" on the border, more unstructured than structured, yet not de-structured; they cannot decide to belong to any official classification, deprived of these letters of nobility. Or, rather, the agency of the letter is not written in a precise way.

We know that the concept of polyphony, elaborated by Mikhail Bakhtin, inspired by Mardi Gras literature, and taken up by Ducrot in linguistics, questions the oneness of the speaking subject. Ducrot (1984) draws a distinction between the speaker, the being who produces an enunciate attributed to it, vs. the subject of the enunciation, which might make several voices speak. It is possible, Ducrot tells us, that some enunciations might not be the product of an individual subjectivity.

In Ducrot's idea of enunciation, voices may appear that are not those of the speaker. These beings that might be expressed through an enunciation, even though no precise words may be attributed to them, Ducrot calls "enunciators". I ask, however, as a counterpart to polyphony, may enunciators exist without a speaker?

When Roussillon (1995) postulated the dual aspect of psychic reality, he tried to answer this question. On the one hand, the psyche concerns experiences that have successfully been inscribed in the representative system, subjected to the functioning of the pleasure—unpleasure principle and of the integration of wish fantasies made conflictual by consideration of reality; on the other hand, the psyche concerns what remains outside the integrative work of the life drives: split-off primary traumatic zones, crypts in search of representations which, being erratic, are subjected to the automatism of repetition. Meanwhile, deadly anxiety is expressed in pure form, as psychosomatic illness, or as repetition compulsion.

I disagree with Ferenczi (1984) when he states that trauma generates an arrest of all psychic activity. This total paralysis, he considers, includes the arrest of perception and at the same time of thought. He adds that it is not possible to defend against an impression that has not been received and postulates that "no memory trace will remain of these impressions, not even in the unconscious, and consequently the origins of the commotion will be inaccessible to memory" (p. 551, translated for this edition).

I understand that Ferenczi is referring to difficulty in calling up remembrance memory. However, I do not think that there is no psychic inscription. Perhaps it is a question of what, in neuroscience, is called implicit memory—that is, sensations lacking representations or emotions that have never been memorized. Freud (1937, p. 260) stated that even things that seem completely forgotten are present somehow and somewhere, and have merely been buried and made inaccessible to the subject. Indeed, it may, as we know, be doubted whether any psychic structure can really be the victim of total destruction. That is to say that he does not consider that no inscription has been produced. The outstanding question is in what way this occurs.

Moreno (2002, p. 43) states that "the subject is affected by what is not represented", and he calls this element an "indeterminate feature without representation". Thus, a feature, according to Moreno, is "pure difference without representation that becomes a mark when a fact gives it meaning." If a feature is to become a mark, he writes, a sanction must transform it into this mark, which separates the unmeaningful from the meaningful. I think that this difference consists in an affect suffered, but since it cannot be represented, it cannot be experienced and, thereby, be bound to a representation. It is as if the person had not been able to become aware of the trace of this feature, to such an extent that, in order to reveal the mark left in the psyche, this person must find a meaning to bind it. The psychic apparatus tries to bind erratic anxiety, and representation is perhaps the most elaborate way to deactivate it. "In dreams we feel no horror that a sphinx is oppressing us, we dream of a sphinx in order to explain the horror we feel," writes Borges (1960). The psychic apparatus does not permit anxiety to remain floating. Anxiety is Pirandellian, as in *Six Characters in Search of an Author* (Pirandello, 1993); anxiety is searching for a representation to which it can be referred as its author. It is for this reason that, in clinical work with traumatic experience, construction takes on the value of interpretation. That is to say that it is not necessarily a search for construction that possesses historical truth, but, rather, it plays a role in the dynamics of the psychic apparatus. Freud (1937) even proposes that the term "reconstruction" should replace the term "interpretation".

It is no longer a question of re-establishing by deduction the original form of the text, as Freud underscored in *Totem and Taboo* (1912– 13) or in *Moses and Monotheism* (1939). Something is missing in a much more radical way: the archaeological metaphor of finding layers unmodified and stratified but perfectly recognizable meets its limit (Press, 2008).

It is less a matter of giving interpretative value to the traumatic scene, the perceptive conformation of which is impossible to ascertain, than of listening to pain awaiting suffering that the subject might finally experience; then, the subject may take the floating enunciate and make it his or her own as an experienced enunciation.

Who is narrating?

In the words of several young girls who had suffered incest, followed up in a centre specializing in outpatient psychotherapy for this complex problem, which I was responsible for coordinating for several years, the traumatic appears (Tesone, 2005) throughout the narration of excitement that had been generated in the girl's body by a burglary: physical stimulation breaking in from the outside without her consent or desire. This body, which responds in an uncontrolled way to external excitation, becomes itself an external body, through a diversification of the ego. This body that made her feel things is not her body. It is a body she does not recognize as her own.

The excitement produced does not, however, make her desirous, since it is de-subjectivizing excitation. It is violence added to the violence of penetration. Desire is not involved; it is excitation stolen from her and a fraud as well, since it triggers drive excitation without the subject's consent. The height of trauma is this brutish and brutal encounter with a de-symbolizing event that does not allow the subject to ensure the continuity of living (Assoun, 1999). The body thereby acquires an extraterritorial quality with a jurisdiction of its own, which requires punishment. It is triply traumatic: due to the burglary and hypercathexis of the act in itself, due to alienating excitation produced without consent or desire, and due to the experience of de-subjectivation that it implies.

It is jouissance associated with the death drive, unbinding of the drives that destructs and annihilates the desiring capacity. The enemy becomes not only the abuser, but also her own body, experienced with shame and even depreciation. It is an abused body that "deserves" punishment for having made her feel excitation in spite of herself, in an uncanny diversification of the ego. As if the girl were to say, "It didn't happen to me; it happened to my body..." An unmetaphorical excitation, pure cathexis, mixed with anxiety, but excitation all the same. The damage is made flesh... in the body. The girl consequently feels disqualified, subjected to an experience not experienced as her own. I consider that, in this clinical work, the analyst's job is not just to lift repression in order to encourage memory and remembering.

As Viderman (1970) suggests, the analyst's task is not to reveal a hidden meaning, but to construct a meaning that was never formed previous to the analytic relation. In the words of Green (1990), the analyst forms an absent meaning. The analyst creates the conditions necessary to enable traumatic experience to be qualified, thought about, experienced, and spoken about, beyond historical truth, but close to experiential truth in its perceptive quality.

The discourse of trauma, as Davoine (1998) points out, is always carried by someone de-subjectivized by knowledge inscribed in the body, to the point that it suspends both attributions judging as well as existence judging. When time is stopped, it is because a subject is needed in order to have time, and in order to have a subject, and, therefore, repression, a succession of signifiers is necessary. In the case of trauma, the chain of signifiers is interrupted, and it is precisely at this place that time is stopped, awaiting a new signifier.

A patient, 35 years old, a professional woman, married, with a 6-year-old boy, tells me after the first interview, in a broken voice, babbling, barely audible, that this is the first time she is able to talk about incest she suffered from her father when she was aged between 7 and 12 years. She said, "I had to construct something in my life; if not, I was afraid I would break down; only now can I talk." Might the devilish monster of traumatic experience appear in the form of the camel's question, "What do you want?" in the novel by the French author, Cazotte (1994), when it queries the fear-struck and also fascinated subject. Like Cazotte's devil in this novel, the devilishly traumatic changes shape, maintaining great ambiguity. Traumatic experience sometimes frightens, but sometimes fascinates. Whether springing from fascination or terror, the effect is the same: muteness. "Small sorrows are loquacious, great ones are mute," as Seneca said (Hippolyte, II, 3, quoted by Montaigne, 1992, p. 8; translated for this edition).

The person risks becoming an enunciate, deprived of enunciation. Even in some cases in which the person is able to speak compulsively of the traumatic experience, sometimes without modesty, this discourse is silenced, or, rather, is full of empty words. In this case, the person is left flabbergasted, trapped in the seduction or terror of traumatic experience, not knowing what to do with it. The subject appears, in the best of cases, when the person is able to take responsibility for doing something different from what was experienced, by de-identifying from this traumatic experience. At the centre mentioned above, the mother of an adolescent girl followed up in psychotherapy as a consequence of incest, who herself had experienced incest, came to the first interview, and when she introduced herself, instead of giving her name, said, "*I am the incested woman.*" The traumatic experience became her identifying introduction instead, negating her identity with her own name. She "was" this enunciate. The damage suffered becomes installed as the paradoxical encysted marrow of an identity emptied of subjectivity. It is similar to what Benyakar (2006) calls the *introduct*—that is, something that remains encysted in the psychic apparatus without representative value. The person "is" the traumatic experience suffered. The person becomes the negative of his or her true subjectivity, oscillating between stifled muteness and Munch's scream, not finding words to tear this suffering out of the interstices of the person's being.

Sometimes, muteness in one language is unshackled in discourse that uses a different language, this passage through language called foreign perhaps facilitating verbal expression. If the subject is to verbalize suffering, to find his or her own voice, the person sometimes calls upon other languages. Far removed from the drive quality implicit in the mother tongue, they are able to express and say in an oblique way what, in the mother tongue, due to excess or deficiency, cannot be put into words: a way to produce languages according to his or her desire, that is, languages of desire.

Luciano, a patient whose mother tongue was Italian, had his analysis with me in French, but sometimes used Italian, in small brushstrokes, as if his discourse were the verbalization of an Impressionist painting. He generally used it to quote phrases he attributed to his mother, as if he had an intra-cavity relationship with her and, at the same time, would have liked to keep her at a distance by having his analysis in French. For a long time, I felt that I had to listen to his few words in Italian within the totality of their drive force, and that the hospitality I gave his words in Italian was more important than the content of associations to which they referred. One day I underscored that he used the Italian language when he was quoting phrases spoken by his mother, as if he wanted me to take care of her directly, in her native tongue. Surprised and anguished in a way I had never perceived before, he added, using a mixture of Italian and French, "Just now I realized that '*mia mamma*' gave me my first kiss on the mouth." He explained that once when he was a child, his mother had passed a piece of candy from her mouth into his, that their tongues had touched in an encounter experienced as never-ending. This anguish, expressed for the first time, could not be said except in Italian, a tongue he had acquired with an excessively incestuous drive quality.

It had to go through a foreign language, in this case French, in order to pacify an excessively intrusive maternal tongue. Through his analysis in

French, which has a different musicality and polysemy, he could express an anguish that, in his mother tongue, burning red-hot, was impossible. This patient would probably never have been able to have analysis directly in his mother tongue, hypercathected with drive quality unspeakable in his native tongue. Through the French tongue, which was also his wife's tongue, he had been able to distance himself unconsciously from the disruptive aspect of a mother tongue whose words burned him, the foreign language thereby acquiring in itself a third-party function. In clinical work on traumatic experience without a subject, the analytic function, after having listened to amorphous material, bits of thought, and snippets of affect, is to make a new film, as proposed by Ferro (2002). I add that it is one in which the analyst scriptwriter may make the unspeakable disruptive experience ("I am the incested woman") capable of figuration and, therefore, of being experienced, so that the first-person singular is no longer the traumatic experience ("I am the incested woman") but, rather, her own ego, rooted in her unconscious but freed from an alienating cystic wrapper. This requires, in Freud's words, the psychic work of construction, "by far the more appropriate description" (1937, p. 261), shared by analysand and analyst, through which disruptive experience may finally be experienced in the first person singular.

The regression habitual in the cure leads us not so much to remembering, as is usual in the analysis of neurotics, but to a zone of representative ambiguity in which representation becomes diffuse and is lost in a cone of shadow. To find it again, or even to produce it, would be the crossroads. However, this construction requires a previous step, which is the deconstruction of what had been acting as a defence—that is, the defensive cyst of non-representation that remains split off as a pure mark awaiting meaning. Construction, in the best of cases, renders the membrane of the cyst porous, and then the affect-representative of the drive breaks through the barrier, entering fluidly into circulation, without reticence, through the chain of unconscious signifiers. The hole in the chain of signifiers is then no longer an empty space aspiring to make nothingness of all meaning, but acts on a new meaning as a motor to construct meaning. In patients subjected to traumatic experience, the narrative ego is emptied of substance, an impersonal voice coming from far away, from some unknown memory or forgetfulness. We do not know who is speaking or to whom the person is speaking. Is it the other in me? Is it the voice of the cyst that replaced it that is speaking? The person searches endlessly for an ego; although it is always essentially dehiscent and unfinished, it may still find harmony with the subject. In order to access its own ego, connected to its conscious and unconscious affects, the narrative must be decanted from a flow of words lost in the haze of emotional–perceptive ambiguity in the defensive cyst. Rather than a monolithic and unmovable tower, the ego agency is like a variable geometric figure in continuous transformation, which, in spite of its polyhedron-like character, with many facets refracting its fragmentary nature, does not define the subject but, instead, places the subject on the axis of emotional responsibility.

Although the analyst is a historian searching not to re-establish historical truth of the facts but, instead, the subject's experiential truth, neither may the analyst completely abandon this search. Even though we know that the search for historical truth is destined to fail, the analyst's intervention cannot be based on a construction totally independent of what is understood of the truth of the facts. It is perhaps necessary to maintain constant tension between the search for historical truth and the mythic construction to preserve it from becoming a meticulously constructed but shaky delusion, to the point that the subject cannot get his or her footing. If not, the analytic process risks acquiring a heavy cathexis of projective suggestion on the analyst's part.

Dreams and dream production may operate then as an equivalent of remembrance. It is through dreams that the subject reappears; their perceptive intensity expresses a form of remembrance of the traumatic experience. "Free association" does not appear in the form of preconscious–conscious association but is freed only as a transaction in dreams, a transaction that acquires the value of remembrance to the extent that the chain of dreams is taken up in the perspective of reconstruction. Sometimes it is through dreams that the patient "remembers", and some of these scenes acquire value as memories of something that occurred.

A female patient, 45 years old, was referred to me by her gynaecologist. His concern, though not the patient's, was that she had never permitted penetration, in spite of having been married for twenty years. Her sexuality had not apparently required this form of expression, and her husband had accepted this. This impossibility would not have been a problem, except that the patient did not allow any gynaecological examination that required penetration, and therefore could not have a pap test or other examinations. Obviously, we did not work on this symptom in a direct manner but, rather, through the patient's free association. Therefore, her sexual life was not an apparent reason for concern. However, after nearly a year in therapy, a dream emerged whose manifest content was the following: "a man took her in a jeep, and then, in a deserted place, something happened that she doesn't remember about the dream". In her associations, she recalls this man, who was a friend of the family, and that one day when she was small, and although she had been in bed with fever, her mother, in her father's absence, had allowed him to take her for a ride in his jeep.

Now, in her adult's eyes, it seemed strange that her mother had accepted something as unusual as letting this man take her for a ride when she was feverish. She remembers a blanket covering her back, but what I am interested in highlighting is not so much the dream images or her associations, so evocative in themselves, but the intense feeling of suffocation and crushing she felt in her body in the dream, a feeling that was not associated with any image, but whose intensity managed to wake her, deeply anguished.

Based on this dream and from the associations that followed, we "reconstructed" what might have happened—that is, the abuse by this man, of which she has no memory. Her feeling in her body and her deep anguish acted, in my opinion, as a trigger to give meaning to her persistent rejection of penetration. Some part of what was disruptive had left a traumatic trace in her, so potentially painful that it led her to absent herself as a subject of pain, an extreme way to avoid it, until, through this and subsequent dreams, we were able to reconstruct what she had probably suffered. When she told her husband the dream and what we had proposed as a hypothesis, he said that he was not surprised, since he had always thought she had suffered some type of abuse. Her difficulty in remembering the fact was associated, in my opinion, not only with the abuse itself, which probably occurred, but to her feeling of orphanhood due to her mother's lack of care; this was an unspeakable pain that lacerated her. Perhaps she preferred to disappear as the subject of abuse, even at the cost of her symptom, rather than to re-experience the iterated pain in her life of orphanhood due to the absence of a mother with her function of protection and caring that every child deserves.

Other situations had made her experience the pain of this absence: as, for example, when she was about 8 years old, she used to have breakfast alone before going to school. For some time, she went to school tipsy, because she began to drink vermouth without eating, which the school finally detected, alerting the family. Her father worked at night and was never present at breakfast time. Many other painful childhood memories emerged, but the most painful had been her actual experience of having been practically "handed over" to a person everybody referred to as "the crazy man". This person, in real life, finally committed suicide.

In this patient, it was not so much the image of the dream but, rather, the intensely experienced bodily feeling that was triggered and operated as an "unremembered" memory at the preconscious–conscious level.

It is as if the regressive current of the psychic apparatus during sleep functioned to trigger an old perception, neither worked through nor integrated, an unmetabolized perceptual force handling of which had remained as if suspended, awaiting the moment to be expressed; the figural quality of the affect-representative in the dream being a substitute for the unthinkable.

We know that in dreams the regressive current allows stimulation of the perceptual pole, precisely the one that, as a consequence of disruptive experience, cannot be expressed spontaneously: it requires a construction. However, reconstruction or construction is always approximate.

As Freud stated about reconstructions (1937, p. 260), they "can often reach only a certain degree of probability". Now, if the construction is the result of a vector of forces determined by the search for perceptual truth of the facts, and the mythical construction of the scene undergone but not experienced by the subject, how do we validate the interest of this construction? We know, as Freud highlights (1937), that it is neither rejection nor conscious validation by the patient that enables us to infer how well grounded the proposed construction might be. Freud considers (p. 265) that in each construction "we do not pretend that an individual construction is anything more than a conjecture which awaits examination, confirmation or rejection". He compares the attitude we should take with respect to effects of the suggested construction to a phrase spoken by a character in a comedy, Nestroy's "Farces", who, to any question or objection, would reply only, "It will all become clear in the course of future developments" (p. 265).

This ironic analogy proposed by Freud has its limits since, obviously, not everything necessarily becomes clear in the course of analysis. As noted by Stoloff (2008), construction, like the work of dream interpretation, meets the limit of what may be known in the unconscious. Just as in dreams, in which meaning escapes us through its navel, there is something like a navel of construction that it is wise to preserve. In construction, the analyst must not pretend to have an all-embracing view of the analysand's unconscious. We would do well to accept that a remnant of unknowable meaning is always left. The challenge is not so much to find the meta-psychological foundation of the construction itself for its validation but, rather, the mutative effect of transformation the construction may achieve *après-coup* or *a posteriori* in the analysand.

In the transference relation of patients who have suffered disruptive experiences, it is particularly advisable to be aware of all the semiotics of figuration, in particular, the intonation of discourse through which we may access the unrepresented—a changing tone of voice as what is figural in sounds of hesitations of lacunar memory of something experienced, but not represented, the voice as a signifier that, through the enunciation of its sound variants, enables it to become a word cathected with affect: it allows passage from a certain affective aphasia to subjectivized discourse and emotions that flow out like a revitalizing thermal spring.

Barthes (1973), in *Le plaisir du texte*, underscores: "With my language I can do everything: even and especially, say nothing. I can do everything with my language, but not with my body. What I hide through my language my body says. I may modulate my message, but not my voice" (p. 45, translated for this edition).

The voice, its timbre, its melody or disharmony, is the least graspable aspect of analytic listening, but sometimes it also allows us to thread together an affect and its possible representation. As the affect gradually emerges, the subject progresses from an impersonal, lifeless, or neutral voice to speaking in a living voice. It is as if the voice were speaking for itself... in representation of the subject, thus acquiring all its meaning—meaning that, as Kristeva (1988) suggests, is found in the register of semiotics.

Words and silence are inseparable in the analytic process, as in poetry, but this is perhaps inherent in the genesis of all aesthetics. From this vantage point, I allow myself to suggest that psychoanalysis, at least in clinical work, is halfway between a conjectural science and a poesis in which the subject appears increasingly in the intonation, harmonious or dissonant, of the drive scansion of the voice, in its prosody, more than in the immobile meaning of an emotionally petrified enunciate. Words become full in so far as they are able to free the concomitant affect from its enclosure.

It is only the appearance of a subject that may finally experience his or her suffering that would make it possible, in the words of Valery (1960), for "the past to have a future" (p. 1526), avoiding deadly repetition compulsion or psychosomatic illness. In this sense, it is naturally not a question of modifying the facts of a traumatic past. Borges (1974, p. 575), the great clinician of the human soul, explained in "The Aleph" that, "to modify the past is not to modify just one fact, it is to cancel its consequences, which tend to be infinite" (translated for this edition).

References

Assoun, P.-L. (1999). *Le préjudice et l'idéal. Pour une clinique sociale du trauma*. Paris: Anthropos.

Barthes, R. (1973). *Le plaisir du texte* [The pleasure of the text]. Paris: Seuil.

Benyakar, M. (2006). *Lo disruptivo*. Buenos Aires: Biblos.

Bion, W. R. (1962). A theory of thinking. *International Journal of Psychoanalysis, 43*: 306–310.

Borges, J. (1960). El hacedor. Ragnarok. In: *Obras completas* (pp. 805–806). Buenos Aires: Emece.

Borges, J. (1974). El Aleph. In: *Obras completas* (pp. 533–629). Buenos Aires: Emece.

Botella, S., & Botella, C. (1992). Le statut métapsychologique de la perception et l'irreprésentable. *Revue Française de Psychanalyse, 56*: 437–457.

Cazotte, J. (1994). *Le diable amoureux*. Paris: Spadem.

Davoine, F. (1998). *El discurso analítico del trauma*. Seminar transcribed from recording, given at the Ministry of Health, Department of Mental Health, Province of Buenos Aires, Argentina.

Ducrot, O. (1984). *Le dire et le dit*. Paris: Minuit.

Duras, M. (1964). *Le ravissement de Lol V. Stein*. Paris: Gallimard.

Ferenczi, S. (1984). Reflexiones sobre el traumatismo. In: *Obras completas* (pp. 545–563). Madrid: Espasa-Calpe.

Ferro, A. (2002). *El psicoanálisis como literatura y terapia*. Buenos Aires: Lumen.

Freud, S. (1912–13). *Totem and Taboo*. In: *Standard Edition, Vol. 13*. London: Hogarth Press.

Freud, S. (1937). Constructions in analysis. In: *Standard Edition, Vol. 23* (pp. 257–269). London: Hogarth Press.

Freud, S. (1939). *Moses and Monotheism*. In: *Standard Edition, Vol. 23* (pp. 7–132). London: Hogarth Press.

Green, A. (1990). *La folie privée*. Paris: Gallimard.

Kristeva, J. (1988). La parole deprimee. In: *La voix. Colloque d'Ivry* (pp. 35–39). Paris: Lysimaque.

Montaigne, M. de (1992). *Essais*. Paris: Arles.

Moreno, J. (2002). *Ser humano*. Buenos Aires: Zorzal.

Pirandello, L. (1993). *Sei personaggi in cerca d'autore* [Six characters in search of an author]. Milano: Tascabili Newton.

Press, J. (2008). Construction avec fin, construction sans fin. *Revue Française de Psychanalyse, 82*: 1269–1337.

Quignard, P. (1998). *Vie secrète*. Paris: Gallimard.

Roussillon, R. (1995). La métapsychologie des processus et la transitionnalité. Rapport au Congrès des Psychanalystes de Langue Française. *Revue Française de Psychanalyse, 59*: 1351–1519.

Stoloff, J.-C. (2008). Les constructions en analyse. Conviction, vraisemblance et changement. *Revue Française de Psychanalyse, 82*: 1533–1541.

Tesone, J.-E. (2005). Incesto. El cuerpo robado. *Revista IDE. Sociedad Brasileira de Psicoanálisis de San Pablo, 41*: 107–114.

Tesone, J.-E. (2009). *A fantasia e o simbólico na cura. Do nao representávelao simbolizável*. Brasilia: Sociedade de Psicanalise de Brasilia.

Valery, P. (1960). *Oeuvres*. Paris: Pleiade.

Viderman, S. (1970). *La construction de l'espace analytique*. Paris: Denoel.

Winnicott, D. W. (1974). La crainte de l'effondrement [Fear of breakdown]. *Nouvelle Revue de Psychanalyse, 11*: 57–63.

Part II

Between completeness and nothingness

7 Could what they say be true?

Assessment of the speech of children and adolescents in case of disclosure of sexual abuse*

It is common that, faced with the revelation of sexual abuse by a child, or even an adolescent, the adult, sometimes paralyzed by the effect of such a revelation, questions the veracity of the child's speech. With doubt creeping into his/her thinking and finds himself unable to determine whether the child is telling "the truth" or if it is mere fantasy speculation, the product of a slightly flowery imagination. How to interpret the speech of a child who trusts an adult, in general a person from his family or school environment, making him a participant in a scene that often lasts for a long time? It seems to me of the utmost importance that the adult is prepared to be able to receive this type of revelation, beyond the ignominious nature of it, without this triggering skepticism or doubt. The opposite would be experienced by the child as a disqualification of his own perception and would therefore contribute to an increase in the trauma so the trauma of sexual abuse would be added to the trauma of adult disbelief.

The moment of revelation is crucial for the psychic future of the child, since the experience of the latter is that with his word, with the revelation of the imposed secret, he is destroying his family—as if it were his speech that destroys the balance, and not the sexual abuse origin of the true trauma. However, unfortunately it is common for doubt to paralyze the adult recipient of the confidence. In a research work carried out in Paris through 300 interviews with professionals in the medical–psycho-social field, it was found that 55% of the interviewees had doubts regarding the veracity of the story of children who complained of having suffered physical or sexual violence within the family, and 13% oscillated between doubt and certainty (Hadjiiski, Agostini, Dardel, & Thouvenin, 1986).

We try here to develop some hypotheses about what raises and enhances this doubt, but above all about its consequences, which lead to an inoperative paralysis in the adult—the product of a tension between the experience in fantasy of the adult and that of the child, and the paralyzing projection of the abuser. With regard to the so-called sexual abuse,

* Published previously in *Abreletras-Psicodiagnóstico*, Ediciones de la Campana, Cátedra de Psicodiagnóstico de la Facultad de Psicología de la Universidad Nacional de La Plata, 1999.

DOI: 10.4324/9781032647791-10

a first level of doubt may be its definition, and it should therefore be specified what we understand by abuse and that it encompasses this notion. If I say misnamed, it is because when we say abuse, we might be assuming that what is prohibited is abuse, but not "use"—a confusion that the term itself generates. If I am punctilious about terminology, it is because words have their importance and are never innocent, and any ambiguity that may generate confusion must be eliminated. For this reason, I prefer to use the term "sexual violence" rather than "abuse", without ignoring that in the Criminal Code of many countries these are considered crimes against sexual integrity. What may seem obvious in our environment as mental health professionals is not evident to other operators in the field of childhood. In this sense it is not redundant to insist that the sexual is not reducible to the sexual organs, but that it supposes giving the sexual all its semantics and complexity, without reducing human sexuality to only its genital aspect or prejudging the place where it can eventually be exercised. From the point of view of the child, sexual violence—as I think it is better to call it—is any act or gesture from which an older person derives sexual gratification. If I speak of violence, it is because all contact of this type involves a certain degree of violence, even if it has not been carried out with physical violence. Violence always exists, at least as psychological violence that provokes psychic effraction and traumatism. These two aspects of violence, physical and sexual, are always inextricably linked, like the reverse and obverse of the two faces of Janus. There is no sexual abuse without violence, just as there is no violence without a certain degree of erogenization. The child cannot semantize what the adult makes them live, and they will not be able to resignify the true traumatic dimension until many years later, through the experience of their own adult sexuality. The traumatic dimension may remain entrenched in a crypt, as apparently outside the psychic life but nevertheless exerting its deleterious effect from the unconscious.

The pleasure sought by the abusive adult is often directly genital (vaginal or anal intercourse, fellatio, masturbation, etc.), but it can also be verbal (sexual terminology) or visual (exhibitionism, pornography, voyeurism, etc.). The essential was summarized by Ferenczi in his famous 1932 article on the confusion of tongues between the adult and the child, where to a request for tenderness and affection on the part of the child, the adult responds with eroticization. The child does not necessarily know that such acts are prohibited, although they often live with guilt—introjected—without becoming aware of the communicating vessels that operate surreptitiously. This guilt does not belong to them: it is the guilt that the abuser does not feel and that they project, without assuming it themselves, into the psyche of the child.

To the trauma of the abuse itself is added another traumatic dimension: the disqualification that the abusing adult makes of the child's own perception by abusing and denying its gravity, thereby subverting all psychic values. Obviously, when the abuse takes place within the family, it acquires a greater gravity, to the extent that it dissolves the primary bonds of affection. There is an erasure of the Oedipal triangle (Tesone, 1994), a confusion of sexes and generations. In a family that we follow in an outpatient psychotherapy center for which I had responsibility in Paris[1], the father had brutally raped his 10-year-old son Antoine (to the point of having caused a skull fracture on one occasion) and had sexually abused his 12-year-old daughter, Lucile, through masturbatory caresses. The scene, repeated over the years, took place in the living room of the family apartment, usually in the presence of the whole family, in front of the TV. This scene, seemingly anodyne in the banality of its repetition, could have been called, in the surreal way, "Portrait of a family in front of the television." The traumatic scene and the anodyne scene overlap, suturing the symbolic and the imaginary with a deadly seam, being suspended in a frozen timelessness. Only when the physical violence of the father was also directed at the mother was the latter finally able to denounce the father to the Justice. The feeling that will predominate in children is that of shame, particularly regarding the experience of their own body. Shame, lived in solitude, is opposed to verbalization: the other should not know. Often the abuser will, through threats and repressive speech, induce in the child the repression of their own speech. The self of the latter, withdrawn, becomes what Ferenczi calls a bipolar ego, made practically of id and super-ego, a self that cannot fulfill the functions that are specific to it: evaluation of the passage of time, location in space, and reality. The process of subjectivation will be gravely mortgaged into a timeless unspeakable. Children are unspeakably fostered by the paradox situation into which they are have been forced: if they speak, they have the feeling that that will make the family explode, if they do not speak, they are condemned to an internal implosion. Stunned, paralyzed in their ability to think and speak, doubting their own perception regarding the gravity of what they experienced, the child will remain silent for a long time. It is for this reason that it is important that when the child finally decides to speak, he or she can be heard by an adult who does not disqualify him/her as to the authenticity of this story. It is a moment of paramount importance for the future of the child. The quality of the adult's listening will depend on whether the abuse ceases, to the extent that it commits the child to denounce the fact, thus avoiding the inexorable traumatic repetition if no external action is involved; and on the other hand, it contributes to reducing the psychic consequences of the fact, giving the child the possibility of trusting an adult. An intervention in this type of situation can never be the isolated action of an adult: it requires a delicate process where several professionals must carry out a coordinated and concerted intervention. A strong network of professionals, involving social workers, teachers, pediatricians, psychologists, psychiatrists, juvenile and criminal judges, as well as substitute families, should support child protection.

At the moment of the removal of the veil from the disruptive scene, during the revelation of the secret and the account of the facts, the adult needs to listen, contain the speech without doubting it, and at the same time maintain a prudent silence. Listening involves focusing your attention on the affections, fears, and anxieties of the child rather than on the facts themselves. To believe in the child's speech is to believe in the affective authenticity of what produces the emergence of that discourse. It consists neither in seeking to establish the truth of the facts nor in questioning them. Its function is not to judge or determine the existence of objectifiable evidence. This will be the function of Justice. The function of the adult is to receive and contain the complaint of the child, to prioritize the word as a privileged mode of exchange.

The dreaded situations of false statements, often invoked to cast doubt on the child's speech, are extremely rare, increasing with age. According to recent studies, they would range between 3% and 8% maximum. This proportion increases, however, in case of divorces, where there may be inducement by one of the parties in conflict. It is known that after having revealed the facts the child has a tendency to retract them, usually due to pressure from the parents themselves. This, known as adaptation and retraction syndrome, occurs in approximately 30% of cases. In countries such as France or Canada, this attitude, far from invalidating the testimony, as would happen in adult justice, reinforces it, considering retraction as being an attitude that singles out the abused child. Of course, the rate of retraction depends not only on the child, but also on the conditions in which the adult listens to his story.

The story of sexual abuse and its listening is disruptive in itself and generates anxiety in both the child and the adult. Everything happens as if sexual violence cannot be thought of, which keeps it out of the field of language. The ignominious, the unthinkable, becomes thinkable. The counter-attitudes of the adult will depend on the echo generated in them by this problem, and in extreme cases it can reveal a fragility that crumbles them. A conflict so deadly in its essence can arouse, in the adult who receives the story, irrepressible affections that alter their representations and their perceptions. The alteration of the latter can induce visual scotomas (when looking at **bruises**, for example), or selective deafness (not hearing, for example, that certain descriptions of sexual scenes cannot be, at a certain age, the pure product of the child's fantasy).

The professional's self may lose its capacity for synthesis. The strangely familiar approximates what Freud described in his article on the sinister, and defensive reactions can lead to maternal's imagos' denial of the authenticity of the story. The need to idealize blood ties, as well as the imagos and paternal functions, alter the perception of listening. In this sense, the discourse of the abused child is subversive, since it questions an established order and denounces the abuse of power of the adult. In the case of the child professional, it questions their ability to understand

and protect them. The abused child disturbs because it reminds adults of the fragility of their own impulsive synthesis under the primacy of the genital, as Freud put it, and reactivates their anxieties in the face of the emergence of partial drives, always chaotic, a repressed base (in the best of cases...), but always present in all adult's drives.

For years the dialectic between ghost and perceptual reality caused a false dilemma, as if one had to choose between one or the other. The ghost, typical of the human, can only be generated from a certain perception, beyond whether it is conscious or unconscious.

When, for example, during a psychotherapy session in our Center, a 5-year-old boy drew a scene of fellatio between a child and an adult, it would have been unwise to think that this was a scene motivated only by a fantastic construction. Most likely, the scene drawn evoked that a child, in his environment or himself (as later confirmed), was being subjected to sexual abuse by an adult.

That in addition, in the drawing, the sex of the adult had an excessive proportion with respect to the size of the child in the same graph, or that the anatomical features or the standing hairs of the adult do not correspond to any real character in his environment, constituted an aggregate phantasmatic construction, which does not invalidate the perceptual base on which it was built. The associations that the child made after the drawing, and certain clarifications regarding the context, made the therapist presume the existence of abuse. But it is not the therapist's role to determine the reality of the fact. It is enough that their strong suspicion leads them to make an intervention through Justice, drawing attention to the presumption of its existence. In the case of which I speak, which did in fact happen, the accusation to Justice was made by me personally, as the medical professional responsible for the Center, after a team meeting and in agreement with the therapist.

I think that psychotherapy cannot be carried out if the therapist suspects the existence of an active, present, and persistent disruptive effect. The ghosts of a child or adolescent should not be worked on psychically, if one is not certain that the disruptive effect has ceased; otherwise, it would be to foster a perverse collusion in the bond.

Finally, I would like to say a few words about the idea of single hearing. In a study done in France it was estimated that, on average, a child who had suffered sexual abuse was forced to repeat the account of the events a dozen times in the course of a trial. From their initial story to the adult they trusted, following with the policeman, or the experts, to the juvenile or criminal judges.

Since it was proven that the repetition of the story is disruptive in itself (what is called secondary victimization), it was sought through the single hearing to avoid the appearance of the child uselessly. This is how it is currently accepted that the interview, with the agreement of the child when they are old enough to do so, is conducted with a childhood specialist and filmed. Subsequently and whenever the child's testimony is subsequently requested, it will refer to the filmed or recorded testimony, and the minor will no longer be subjected to a new and repeated appearance, which could go as far as an oral trial, in the case of a criminal instance. In recent years, use has been made of the Gesell Chamber[2], but it is not the same. This is a controversial and questionable procedure, since it does not respect the necessary privacy of any psychological interview with a young child, carried out by a professional in the field of psychology, whose function is to create a climate of trust and security in the interview and not be subjected to the simultaneous interrogation of representatives of the Judiciary or of the lawyers of the parties, who sometimes ask questions vi written messages during the course of the interview. In short, I allow myself to insist on the importance of not questioning the veracity of the child's speech, but accepting its verisimilitude, holding on to the affective authenticity of the story it generates. This is the best way to restore the value of verbalization—a step prior to any attempt to elaborate the traumatic and to allow the child to emerge from the crushing of the symbolic into which they have been compelled: to finally be able to think the unthinkable, the unthinkable being listened to, even if it is the dark side of the human being.

Notes

1 Centre Médico-Psycho-Pédagogique E. Pichon-Rivière—9 Cour des Petites-Ecuries, 75010 Paris.
2 A Gesell chamber is a space separated into two rooms, divided by a one-way mirror that allows the observer to watch what is happening in the other half of the room, but not vice versa.

References

Hadjiiski, E., Agostini, D., Dardel, F., & Thouvenin, C. (1986). *Du cri au silence. Contribution à l'étude des attitudes des intervenants médico-sociaux face à l'enfant victime de mauvais traitements.* Paris: C.T.N.E.R.H.I.

Ferenczi, S. (1932). Confusion of tongues *between* adults and the child. *International Journal of Psychoanalysis, 30* (No. 4, 1949): 225–230.

Tesone, J. E. (1994). Notas psicoanalíticas sobre el incesto consumado. El triángulo deshecho? *Revista de Psicología y Psicoterapia de Grupo, Buenos Aires, 17* (1).

8   The importance of the No in the prevention of sexual violence against children and adolescents*

For a long time, the true dimension of this problem has been disregarded, as little reliable statistical data has been available in many countries. It was presumed that sexual violence against children was limited to some isolated pedophiles, without considering the seriousness of true pedophile networks, to the dissemination of which the Internet has contributed. The so-called grooming, of dangerous diffusion on the internet, consists of the recruitment of a minor by an adult with a false identity, who pretends to be a minor. Networks include the marketing of pornographic material, including children, and the increasing numbers of the euphemistically called "sex tourism" pedophiles.

Problematic, but not devoid of an effect of fascination for some media, it is judged and condemned, but not analyzed. It is useful to quantify its existence. The first French survey on sexual abuse suffered by children was commissioned in 1989 by the Ministry of Health. It was conducted on a representative sample of the 18–60 year-old population, of whom 6.2% reported having been victims of sexual abuse in their childhood: 7.8% were women and 4.5% men. Most sexual violence occurred at puberty for both sexes. Half of the first abuses happened before age 12 for boys and before age 11 for girls. Abusers were, in 63% of cases, people known to the victim, and in 17% of cases they were part of the family. The disclosure of abuse at the time it occurred existed in only one case out of 3. The repetition of abuse for the same person was cited by 0.8% of men and 3.2% of women. Of the latter, 4% had been victims of incest. It is highlighted in the survey that there were no differences between the various social classes.

D. Finkelhor, a pediatrician who works in the United States and has acquired more experience in this field, concludes in a 1994 article that epidemiological surveys conducted in some 24 countries show that "sexual abuse is a real danger for 5 to 20% of all children, girls having between 2 and 3 times more risks than boys" (Finkelhor, 1994). A recent survey

---

* A summary of this text was published as, "Is sex education possible?", in the Buenos Aires newspaper *La Nación*, November 22, 2004.

DOI: 10.4324/9781032647791-11

carried out in Argentina, within the framework of a joint research project between a team of researchers from the Faculty of Psychology of the National University of Mar del Plata (Mosteirin & Tesone, 2003), has made it possible to quantify the seriousness of the problem.

This survey on adolescent health indicators was presented to a representative sample of adolescents enrolled in the third year of polymodal public and private schools in the city of Mar del Plata, in the form of a previously standardized anonymous self-questionnaire. It shows that 14.5% of the adolescents surveyed say they had suffered sexual abuse during their childhood. Of these, 84% are female adolescents and 16% are male adolescents. Of the young people abused, 0.5% of boys and 1.7% of adolescents were abused by a close relative. Only 3% of abused boys and 16.7% of abused girls were able to talk about it with anyone. In other words, it can be said that denial, rejection, and silencing continues to prevail in society in relation to this problem

The sexual abuse of a child or adolescent is, first and foremost, a gesture of violence. Whether or not it is accompanied by physical violence, we always find the existence of psychic violence. Like the god Janus of Greek mythology, they are the two inseparable faces of abuse. We prefer the term "sexual violence" to "sexual abuse," because the latter is ambiguous—a confusion to which Argentina's penal code contributed by, until recently, qualifying sexual abuse as "indecent assault"—as if there could be an abuse that is not.

Coercion towards the child can be exercised by force, intimidation, blackmail, or seduction (which often acquires a hypnotic dimension)—generally, through any form of pressure from a person who is older than the child. No child is exempt from this risk. Sexual violence against minors is any act or gesture through which an older person derives sexual enjoyment.

In no case should the existence of a "mutual consent" be mentioned, since the child, given his physical and mental immaturity, is in no position to give free consent. The adult responds perversely with the language of eroticization to the child's request for love and tenderness, considering him not as a being, but as an object at the service of his own enjoyment. This act has the consequence of generating a psychic injury traumatic effect of which can manifest itself immediately in the form of psychopathological symptoms of childhood—depression, suicide attempts, encopresis, learning disorders, anorexia, bulimia, etc.—which may emerge, many years later, in adulthood, as a real time bomb. In the experiences of the abused person, feelings of guilt, shame of their own body, devaluation, and self-harm prevail. In the abuser, the most frequent is denial and the absence of guilt.

Faced with the horror and magnitude of this phenomenon, is it possible to take preventiven action? How can one help a child to protect himself from this type of bullying, so that he can, as far as possible, feel entitled to say no? Without falling into the simplicity of thinking that the simple cannot, by itself, in an accurate way prevent violence, it is the first step of all preventive action. What would be the most appropriate way? The answer is not simple and deserves a prior analysis.

Parents, educational institutions, and, in time, society often demand that the child should, from earliest childhood on, respond affirmatively to the proposals of the adult. The adult expects a "yes" from the child, based on the educational principles that we have inherited from the century of enlightenment and religions. It thus responds to an educational ideal that places the adult on an omniscient pedestal, as the remnant of the figure of the *pater familias* inherited from Roman times, and, as such, with arbitrary power of life and death over the child, the legal status of the latter being equivalent to that of the slave. The conception of the child as a subject of law is a recent appearance in the history of mankind. Concomitantly, the child is considered someone capable of a valid story for justice to consider his testimony.

This is how the story of the child is valued in all its dimension of plausibility by a large part of the laws in force in European countries, in Canada, and, increasingly, in the Argentine Courts. Sexual violence is one of the greatest abuses that a child can suffer. Such stories appear regularly in the media, driven either by cases of abuse of public notoriety and/or as a result of court cases. Between condemnation and fascination, between denial and unhealthy insistence, it is rare that these cases are spoken of in a sensible way. An unspeakable problem for many, it becomes unthinkable, thus making it difficult to devise protection programs that benefit children.

Society reacts in a scandalized, visceral way, not giving space for a real debate on the best way to avoid abuse or, if it has occurred, to lessen its traumatic effect on the child. Talking composedly about sexuality remains taboo, even in the twenty-first century: it is not talked about—or, rather, talked about too much, but inadequately. The aforementioned controversial sex education courses in schools have been tested for different purposes. This has undoubtedly been an advance over the ignorance that came with avoiding talking about sexuality. But these courses, even in the best cases, provide information on the physiological functioning of the sexual and reproductive organs, or on sexual diversity—which is, incidentally, necessary—but they do not give tools for the prevention of sexual violence. The program for the prevention of sexual violence against children used in Canada, and later taken up by the French Ministry of Health, is based on making the child aware that their body belongs to them, and that no one can use it for their own interest. Via video, graphic material, and ongoing dialogue with children, the abovementioned programs highlight the rights of the child not to submit to the adult who proposes such acts. It supports the firm conviction that the child must be informed of their inalienable right to reject the perverse proposal of the abuser, emphasizing that the law and institutions guarantee it. The child is thus legitimized in their right to say no to an adult if the proposal attacks of their condition as a person. It is essential that the child feels validated by the adults in whom they trust that their body is their body and that it belongs only to them. It is worth insisting that the sexual abuse of a child is not only of their body: it is, above all, an abuse of their person, a greater attack on their own subjectivity in becoming. While it is their body that initially pays tribute, it is their entire identity that gets caught up in the cartography of the sexual language of the abusing adult. The latter tries to paralyze the child in their own ability to think and coerces them into silence and isolation. Now, how can a child be encouraged to reject the perverse proposal of an adult who intends to abuse their body, if they have not previously been legitimized in their right to say no in other circumstances? If they have been educated in submission to a logic that presupposes that the adult can impose their will *per se*, by their mere condition as an adult, without considering that the condition of adult is not synonymous with psychic balance?

Teaching a child their legitimacy to reject such proposals can, however, only be achieved in a social context of citizen freedom and democracy. Having control over the body of the other has always been the way of totalitarian, public, private or corporate systems. For this reason, it is crucial that democratic systems foster in children, through education and prevention programs, the possibility of exercising the right to say no, a condition that is not sufficient, but necessary to protect children and promote in children their own capacity for care. The latter implies that the adult, who is in a position to protect them from the perversity of the abuser, can take into account the child's story, particularly at the crucial moment of the revelation of the abuse. Consequently, it requires the institutions that deal with children to admit that when any of their members breaks the social contract of respect for children, it is essential that they be judged and not seek to inadequately protect themselves by way of a corporatist logic. At stake is the mental health of children—and concomitantly, what is no less serious: the credibility of the institutions on which the symbolic law of the social contract is based.

References

Finkelhor, D. (1994). Abus sexuel et santé sexuelle chez l'enfant. Nouveaux dilemmes pour le pédiatre [Sexual abuse and sexual health in children: New dilemmas for the pediatrician]. *Schweizerische Medizinische Wochenschrift, 124* (51–52): 2320–2330.

Ministry of Health, France (1989). Abus sexuels à l'égard des enfants [Sexual abuse of children]. Dossier technique du Ministère de la Solidarité, de la Sante et de la protection sociale, sous la direction de M. Gabel, Paris.

Mosteirín, C., & Tesone, J. E. (2003). Investigation research. Faculty of Psychology, National University of Mar del Plata, Argentine: Fac. de Psicología, UNMDP.

9   Femicide and orphanhood*

Femicide leaves one or more children orphaned by the mother, as is evident. This situation is disruptive and traumatogenic in itself, not only because of the loss of the mother, but also because of the circumstances in which said loss occurs. The child is stunned and paralyzed in his or her ability to think and elaborate what happened. Orphanhood, however, concerns both parents, since by killing the mother, the father abrogates his paternal function, which falls into an abyss from which it can no longer recover.

The child will continue to have one biological parent, eventually in prison, but definitively loses that parent in his symbolic role. In the act of murdering the mother, the father simultaneously murders the paternal function. He therefore commits a triple crime: against the mother's body, the paternal function, and the inner representation of the symbolic father as primary caregiver of the child. The child is deprived of both parents and remains in affectively open, in solitude, facing of their own impulses without anyone to contain them and able to provide them with a structuring metabolization of their fears and anxieties. Sometimes a fourth death is also added, if, having committed such an aberrant crime, the father commits suicide. From my point of view, the murder of the mother is, at the same time, a form of filicide. It kills in the child not only the real mother, but the caring ability of the inner parents. To the helplessness of orphanhood must be added the violence of having witnessed, either as an eyewitness or even as an auditory witness, later, to the murder of the mother. Having witnessed such violence has a deleterious effect on the child's psychic life, the magnitude of which is difficult to measure. It can have an immediate implosion effect, through which the child is stunned, paralyzed in the ability to think, but simultaneously, like a time bomb, continuing acting in silence, in a timeless way, as if it were an anti-personnel bomb in their unconscious, which continues to dynamite their personality into advanced stages of life.

* Conference within the framework of the Table-Debate, "Femicide: A Current Problem", Honorable Chamber of Deputies of the Nation, Buenos Aires, November 25, 2016.

DOI: 10.4324/9781032647791-12

The violence, which is rarely unexpected but is the culmination of a long anticipatory process, could have been inscribed directly on the child's body or passively suffered as a silent witness to violence between parents, particularly, in the case of femicide, by the father towards the mother. The child not only lives terrified that this violence will turn against them, and fearing for their lives, they rightly despair because of the violence of the father towards their mother. They fear the death of the mother and/or their own and try unsuccessfully protect themselves. If the crime materializes, they can experience it as a personal failure for not having managed to avoid it, a source of guilt and self-reproach.

This inscription of violence can destroy the child's inner world, leaving them in complete helplessness in the face of their own impulses. One of the functions of parenting is to contain and metabolize the violence of children, to host it through affection. If violence is something inherent to the human being, the way out is not by denying it, but by containing, channeling, or deactivating it, offering a symbolic outlet to its manifestation. Thus, it can become something creative, which allows a regulated direct impulse discharge or, in a sublimated way, in the form of literary, musical, or manual activities or other interests. The important thing in order to live in a civilized way is to have the ability to renounce a drive discharge to the gross state and to orient it creatively for oneself and for the social group. It is the basis of the social contract of which Rousseau spoke, and which Freud described in *Civilization and Its Discontents* (1930, p. 59).

The renunciation of the direct satisfaction of aggressive impulses is the precondition that must be paid as an inescapable contribution of each one in order to be able to live in society. The family group is, beyond its configuration, the first experience of life in society. There the child feels, for the first time, as in a true melting pot, all human emotions. Outside this contract, which supposes that all people accept and integrate it, violence is unleashed in a speculative, uncontrollable way, in a deadly spiral, which can lead to tragedy.

The child, because of immaturity and their developing personality, is particularly exposed to the psychic implications of the outbreak of violence. It is almost more their psyche that fragments and suffers terrible— sometimes irreparable—damage than the tribute their body can pay with the marks of violence. There is no natural essence that defines man or woman, but strongly epochal cultural determinants and tributaries of the dominant culture. Children need to be able to identify with the adults who raise, care for, and educate them, regardless of gender.

The *princeps* function of the family, beyond its configuration, is to produce alterity—that is, that the child is respected as a subject and is provided with the bases to build their own subjectivity. Biological parents, or those who fulfill the function of parenting, operate as models with which the child will identify, consciously or unconsciously. If the paternal model is one of violence, the problem can be repeated transgenerationally, since the identification mechanisms occurs unconsciously. This child may, in turn, be violent with others, either their peers or, later, the other, the non-self, whose paradigm par excellence for the male represents the woman.

Man has to be feminine enough, that is, to admit the psychic bisexuality existing in every human being, to live in peace with his own masculinity. Chauvinism is often the denial of the feminine in men, and their violent reaction towards women is a way of wanting to push aside the feminine in themselves. A manifestation of impotence is, in the face of the enigma that women represent for men, a symbol of the foreignness of everyone else. The other is always irreducible to one's fantasies, and to accept the foreignness of that other is also to accept the part of one's own foreignness in oneself—that is, the unconscious. Violence can be a desperate attempt to annul the irreducible foreignness of the other, to pretend that this feminine other is a controllable and manipulatable possession, according to the craziest fantasies, as if the woman were a fetish object.

I want to emphasize that every child has the right to be loved, cared for, educated, contained, and accompanied during childhood. The human being is the living being who requires external care for the longest time. This function of care is, ideally, exercised by the biological parents, but if they cannot fully assume this function, it is not advisable to sacralize blood ties. The family is, first and foremost, a cultural institution. If the father or partner of the mother has, by murdering the mother, renounced his paternal function, others, then either someone from the extended family of the children, or adoptive or foster families will be able to provide the child with what he or she needs from the adult: affection, care, containment.

To which must be added a psychological follow-up of children as a highly recommended proposal to help them metabolize the incalculable disruptive effect suffered, so that it does not become entrenched in their psyche and continue, from the bottom of their unconscious, to exert a traumatogenic effect on their subjectivity—hence the limits of the much-sought family reunification imposed, not without certain candidness, by some judges who sacralize blood ties to the detriment of the mental health of the child. Femicide is a tragedy for the condition of women, but it is, simultaneously, a tragedy for children who live with the man who has attacked them, either directly or through an intermediary, in the figure of the mother.

Reference

Freud, S. (1930). *Civilization and Its Discontents. Standard Edition, Vol. 21*. London: Hogarth Press.

10 The divine jouissance, the feminine position, and the mystics*

"What does a woman want?" asks Freud (in Jones, 1953, p. 421), while comparing it to an unexplored continent—an enigma that he left unresolved, without ever having revealed it, a question that may seem unusual for times in which we are no longer supposed to know whether it is a woman or a man or whether it is femininity or masculinity?

Solving such riddles has not brought much luck to the daring that plunged into the abyss of answers, whether contemplating Oedipus in front of the Sphinx or Tiresias in front of Athens. I will advance, however—not without apprehension, in the reformulation of the question—proposing to travel together on the path that leads us to approach a possible answer, knowing in advance that it is advisable to take the precaution of not trying to find a univocal answer.

Tiresias, before being a fortune teller, was a woman, at least for a certain time. As a result of having beaten, or injured, or killed—in any case, separated—two copulating snakes, he lived in a woman's body. Later, attacking a pair of snakes again, he become a man again. His passage through the feminine condition gave him the experience of both sexes.

Now, one day, Zeus argued with Hera and affirmed that, during the sexual act, the woman achieved greater pleasure, while Hera maintained the opposite; so they decided to consult Tiresias, since she was the only one who had known the two conditions. To the question that was put to him, he replied that, if there were ten parts of pleasure, the man enjoyed only one while the woman enjoyed nine times. Hera reacts furiously to this response and turns Tiresias into a blind man, while Zeus, satisfied with the answer, makes him a fortune teller. Hera's passionate reaction is paradoxical.

Nicole Loraux (1989) stresses that women's secrets must definitely remain well guarded. The blind eyes of the Theban show that he no longer

* Published in the *Journal of the Argentine Psychoanalytic Association*, Vol. 66, No. 3, September 2009, Buenos Aires; and in the *Revista Brasileira de Psicanálise*, Vol. 42, No. 4, pp. 139–143, Sao Paulo, December 2008. (Modified version of an article published in *Revue Française de Psychanalyse*, Vol. 70, December 2006.)

DOI: 10.4324/9781032647791-13

has a need to see... since he knows. But he had to pay a heavy tribute for having valued the enjoyment of women. Should such enjoyment remain silent?

Classically the feminine has been culturally more linked to suffering or *hysterical belle indifference* than to enjoyment, whether this applies to the pains of childbirth, the rules, the hysterical frigidity or the masochism, called feminine.

Lacan (1975) had the merit of subverting this commonplace, proposing that the woman, in relation to what she designates as enjoyment in the phallic function, has an "additional" enjoyment, adhering perhaps to the affirmation of Tiresias. He affirms: "I believe in the enjoyment of women as long as they are in more." And he remarks that this enjoyment is even more evident in the excess of mystics, of which the face in ecstasy of Saint Teresa, immortalized in the statue of Bernini in the church of Santa Maria della Victoria in Rome, is a paradigmatic example. But even there feminine enjoyment must remain veiled, even for the saint: "it is clear that the essential testimony of the mystics is precisely to say that they feel it, but that they know nothing about it." They have to pretend to ignore the enjoyment lived or, at least, that it does not transcend.

As Marie-Christine Laznik (1990) recalls, for Lacan, sexuation depends on the relationship that human subjects have with the phallic question and what they point to in their desire. For Lacan, real sex is not decisive for a subject with respect to the side he will come to occupy in the formula. This statement by Lacan, which maintains a certain ambiguity, has the merit of underlining that the feminine can be before a position, not necessarily linked to anatomical sex. This author affirms that St. John of the Cross was on the female side. Did he not he write "in the feminine gender" to the extent that the nuptial symbolic feminizes the discourse? St. John of the Cross refers to God, addressing God as the bridegroom:

Where did you hide, Beloved, and left me groaning?
Like the deer you fled,
Having wounded me,
I went after you, crying, and you were gone.

O forests and thickets,
Planted by the hand of the Beloved!
O vegetable meadow,
Glazed flowers!
Say if it has happened to you.

(San Juan de la Cruz, 1991a)

Freud made femininity the "bedrock of both sexes" (1937, p. 252). Although, as Christian David (1992) points out, psychic bisexuality in men is not symmetrical with psychic bisexuality in women.

The discourses of the mystics unfold in full paradox. From their narcissistic omnipotence, they seek to make One greater than oneself—that is, with God, sometimes in retreat, sometimes in a fusional impulse. In a specular relationship they seek narcissistic completeness by simultaneously generating a detachment that "excenters" them from themselves. Saint Teresa de Jesus (1997) begins one of her poems this way:

I live, without living in me.

As Didier Anzieu (1980) points out, the nucleus of being is found not in the center, but in its periphery, where God surrounds it:

I am yours, for you brought me up,
Yours, for you redeemed me,
Yours, therefore you suffered me,
Yours for you called,
Yours because you waited for me,
Yours, for I did not miss:
What do you send of me?

Can God be an object choice? If, as Winnicott (1951) emphasizes, every object choice is a created-found object, God cannot be an object, however grandiose, since he leaves no room to create it. He simply Is, to such an extent that humans cannot even name Him. He is who Is.

At most, it is the quality of subjective, narcissistic object implied by this choice that can be highlighted. In mystical love, we find ourselves in the middle of the oceanic feeling of which Freud spoke in *Civilization and Its Discontents* (1930) which needs to return to a state prior to that of the distinction between a self and a non-self, as is characteristic of primary narcissism. However, as Laznik points out, instead of resorting to a primary mother, it is to the nostalgia of the father that Freud attributes the feeling of making One with the great All.

In this approach to God, the mystic pays the price of a self-detachment, of a de-subjectivation that marks his abolition as a subject. It lives only through the flashes of the object, brilliance that illuminates… simultaneously veiling (barely) the carnal pleasure of ecstasy. This enjoyment must remain unknown or at least veiled to others. If the veil were to fall, enjoyment would acquire legitimacy through religious ablativity. Consequently, the mystic enjoys… without sin and without reproach, sheltered from all eyes, in the monastic cloister.

The narcissistic ego, linked to the narcissism of death, says Green (1983), must fight both against its impulses and against the object, both always traumatic for the human being. Faced with this combat that every subject must perform, the narcissist pretends to be accepted, choosing a narcissistic, arrogant, and deceptive isolation. They desperately seek the flattening of desire, the neutral, and the distance of the object.

The mystic, in full paradox, represses the drives through an affective perversity that avoids, hesitantly, the direct satisfaction of the drives, but does not totally renounce them. As for the object, they do not reject it, do not put it at a distance; they enter into a specular relationship in which the gaze attributed to God divinizes it and confirms it in its narcissistic omnipotence. United with God, Anzieu (1980) remarks, the mystic participates in divine creation and continues it. In mystical union the whole soul becomes the other: "Loved with beloved, loved in the Beloved transformed."

The libidinal burden is strongly genitalized: Jesus Christ is the divine Bridegroom, the church his Bride. This libidinal recharge endows the mystic "with an exceptional energy that allows him to face loneliness, the weather, the desert, persecutions or consecrate himself to the foundation of multiple confraternities or monasteries. But the experience of fullness requires the conjunction of two elements: libidinal superabundance and access to the feeling of a primary and limitless Self" (Anzieu, 1980)—the paradox of finding the full in the extreme void.

Bataille (1957) reminds us that human beings are discontinuous—that, between one being and another, there is an abyss, a discontinuity. He defines eroticism as the attempt to annul this discontinuity: "what is at stake in eroticism is always the dissolution of constituted forms." Bataille proposes three forms of eroticism: that of bodies, that of hearts, and the sacred, which contains all three. This eroticism, divine or sacred, is the search for the full, unlimited being, which no longer limits personal discontinuity. Bataille emphasizes that what characterizes mystical experience is an absence of object: a choice that is not devoid of a relative death sentence of subjectivity. Movement that emphasizes that death is at stake in every erotic search. The expression *"petite mort"* with which the French language describes the experience of orgasm is eloquent regarding the provisional loss of subjectivity that every sexual encounter produces. It is this search for de-subjectivation that, in the mystic, becomes extreme paroxysm and ecstasy:

> I live without living in me.
> and in such a way I hope
> that I die because I do not die.
>
> (San Juan de la Cruz, 1991b)

The field of eroticism, says Bataille, is that of the transgression of prohibitions, the desire that triumphs over the forbidden. It links erotic experience to holiness without making them equivalent. Its point of convergence is intensity. In mystics there is transgression, particularly of boundaries, and a perceptible libidinal charge in the enjoyment of ecstasy. But the sacred condition demands that enjoyment remain veiled, in the name of that greater than oneself. St. Teresa de Jesus (2000) said that "even if hell should sink her, she could not, but persevere."

Persevere in what? Would it not be in righteous enjoyment, even if it is divine, and beyond that it can lead her to hell? Enjoy also in suffering, often associated, by identification, with the pain of Christ crucified. In any case, it is a question of a shift in the limit that allows obtaining enjoyment, of which the prayer and the stages of the dwellings of the soul of Saint Teresa are a good example. Only in the seventh and final resting place does she accede to "communion-union":

> "God's ultimate habitation in the soul takes place in this dwelling place. Although, to tell the truth, total and perfect communion only occurs in the afterlife.
>
> When it happens for the first time, Christ appears, visible in the eyes of the soul, with great radiance, beauty and majesty, as after the risen one, and tells the soul that it is time for it to take its own things, for he will take care of his.
>
> It gives the impression at that moment that God gives a foretaste of all the joy, joy, and peace of heaven. There are no words or comparisons to describe what is lived. The union of God and smallness is realized, like a drop of water in the immensity of the ocean."
>
> (Santa Teresa de Jesús, 2000)

Rosolato (1980 proposes that ecstasy is a sublimated transposition of sexual orgasmic enjoyment, which exalts all visions of sacred union, such as the "Song of Songs", in a narcissistic unfolding of a symmetrical nature. Rosolato quotes El Halladj to underline this mirror relationship: "The eye through which you see me is the eye through which I see you."

What link could we try to establish between Tiresias, feminine enjoyment, mystics, and choice of object?

Lavie (1980) points out that the mystic gives himself the right of the common shamelessness that habitually makes others hide their source of enjoyment. The mystic is convinced that God "sanctifies" everything, or at least that one can do in His name what could not otherwise be done with impunity. God would then be an object-non-object linked to a subject that would not be such, but would be One, in that communion-union of which St. Teresa spoke.

Through this detour, mystics feel liberated from what they live, as if the libidinal burden came to them innocently:

> I entered where I didn't know
> and stayed not knowing,
> all knowledge there transcending.

I didn't know where I was,
but I saw myself there
not knowing where I was.
Great things I understood
I can't say what I felt
since I didn't know,
all knowledge there transcending.

(San Juan de la Cruz, 1991b)

As Hamon (1980) remarks, a lexicon is imposed: "dilation" as opposed to "dryness," "softness," "favors," "delicious wounds," "earthly pleasures," "rapture," "transports," the "theft of the spirit," "wounds of love," between "ecstasy" and "suspension" and "tasty torments." Enjoyment is explicitly referred to the body: "The body does indeed have its share of happiness and delights, very noticeably...", confesses Saint Teresa of Avila. She emphasizes to the extreme, Hamon suggests, the sensations: grasping, rigidity of the limbs or disarticulation of the whole body, weakening of the pulse, loss of breath, fainting and levitations; not counting the images of liquefaction, or penetration.

Through centuries of male domination, female enjoyment has not been readily admitted—a prohibition of which hysterics were the main victims. They were the victims of such intolerance, paying a heavy price, sometimes at the cost of their own lives at the stake of the Inquisition. Even today, mutilation-excision of the clitoris is practiced on girls in vast areas of the world, condemning women to not obtaining the pleasure that this organ normally gives them.

What if the discourse of the mystics showed—in an extreme way, although veiled by religious demands—the additional enjoyment of women, otherwise unspeakable if one does not want to suffer the same punishment as Tiresias?

References

Anzieu, D. (1980). Du code et du corps mystiques et de leurs paradoxes. *Nouvelle Revue de Psychanalyse, 22.*

Bataille, G. (1957). *L'érotisme.* Paris: Edition de Minuit.

David, C. (1992). *La bisexualité psychique,* Paris: Payot.

Freud, S. (1930). *Civilization and Its Discontents. Standard Edition, Vol. 21.* London: Hogarth Press.

Freud, S. (1937). Analysis terminable and interminable. *Standard Edition, Vol. 23.* London: Hogarth Press, 1964.

Green, A. (1983). *Narcissisme de vie, narcissisme de mor.* Paris: Editions de Minuit.

Hamon, M.-C. (1980). Le sexe des mystiques. *Ornicar?,* 20–21: 159–180.

Jones, E. (1953). *Sigmund Freud: Life and Work, Vol. 2.* London: Hogarth Press.

Lacan, J. (1975). *Le séminaire Encore, Livre XX.* Paris: Seuil.

Lavie, J.-C. (1980). Servir. *Nouvelle Revue de Psychanalyse, 22.*

Laznik, M.-C. (1990). La mise en place du concept de jouissance chez Lacan. *Revue Française de Psychanalyse, 1* (54): 55–82.

Loraux, N. (1989). *Les expériences de Tirésias. Le féminin et l'homme grec.* Paris: Gallimard.

Rosolato, G. (1980). Présente mystique. *Nouvelle Revue de Psychanalyse, 22.*

San Juan de la Cruz (1991a). *Cántico espiritual, canciones entre el alma y el esposo.Obra completa.* Madrid: Alianza Editorial.

San Juan de la Cruz (1991b). *Noche oscura, cántico espiritual. Obra completa.* Madrid: Alianza Editorial.

Santa Teresa de Jesus (1997). *El libro de la vida. Complete works.* Burgos: Monte Carmelo.

Santa Teresa de Jesus (2000). *Se trata de amar mucho.* Buenos Aires: Paulinas.

Winnicott, D. W. (1951). Transitional objects and transitional phenomena. In: *Through Paediatrics to Psycho-Analysis.* London: Hogarth Press, 1975.

11   Masculinities checkmated?*

Masculinity, even in the plural, is a concept that would needs a definition before one can debate whether or not it is in check. Masculine–feminine; male–female; father–mother: they are strongly epochal concepts that intersect and slide into each other, like Russian dolls, often embedded. The idea would be like running away from an a-historical essentialism.

Freud initially defined masculine as active and feminine as passive, although later, speaking of human sexuality, he spoke about psychic bisexuality in both sexes; there are therefore active and passive attitudes in both. Lacan (1975) introduced the famous formula of sexuation, in which he emphasized that man could occupy a feminine place; he quoted Saint John of the Cross, who, in his poems, occupied a feminine place when facing God—but this did arise out of binarism. Volnovich and Rodulfo (1997) suggest deconstructing the phallocentric scaffolding of psychoanalysis, since the primacy of the phallus lives on binarism.

This classic binary is currently strongly questioned, not only by gender studies movements of self-designated sexual identity, but also by LG-BTQ+ movements. Psychoanalytic theory also requires a reformulation of its theory, which tends to rely more on the complex thinking of Edgar Morin (1914), on Derrida's theory of deconstruction (1967), or on Deleuze's rhizomatic (Deleuze & Guattari, 1976) than on classical binarism. We are far from Napoleon's assertion, taken up by Freud, that anatomy is destiny.

The history of sexuality is a discontinuous story that is impossible to tell in terms of a line of progression from the most implacable repressions to the most complete emancipations. If we were to underline a single index of the new order, we could take the anachronism into which virginity has fallen as a value. Gender identity does not coincide with the anatomical condition of male or female. Currently, in Germany, it exists in the forms issued by the public administration: under the category of gender, one can

* Conference within the framework of a panel held at Freud's Bar, DAIN Usina Cultural, Nicaragua 4899, Buenos Aires, November 8, 2019, organized by the Argentine Psychoanalytic Association.

DOI: 10.4324/9781032647791-14

put, man, woman or neutral. In many kindergartens in Sweden, teachers refer to children in the neutral gender.

Currently, in Argentina, many young people advocate for an inclusive language that leaves gender in an indefiniteness lived as freedom in choice. A small detour through history can clarify some concepts according to time or culture. The word "homosexuality" would have appeared in the Occident in 1869, and the word "heterosexuality" in 1890. In ancient Greece and Rome, there was no notion of heterosexuality and homosexuality: they distinguished activity from passivity, opposed the phallus [*fascinus*] to all orifices [*spintrias*] (Quignard, 1994). Greek pederasty was a rite of social passage. By ritual sodomization, the adult's sperm transmitted virility to the adolescent. There was no change of roles. The penetration of the passive adolescent, *éromene*, by the active adult, *eraste*, was an obligatory passage of the transmission of virility in warrior Sparta. The meaning of the passage was to take the pubescent away from the passivity of the gynoecium and to make a warrior, a breeder, a father, and a citizen. For the Greeks, virtue meant sexual potency. Manhood was the duty of the free man, the mark of his potency. The only model of Roman sexuality was the domination of the dominated over all others. The slave could not sodomize his master, but the reverse could happen.

The very notion of chastity bore surprising edges. Chastity was the integrity of the caste, of the embryo carried by the woman, but whose fecundity depended in the Roman imaginary about virile sperm. Nothing is less chaste than this form of chastity: the woman could have relations with other men when she was pregnant, since filiation was not at risk. Pleasure does not have to be faithful; the valuable thing was to preserve the filiation. Roman marriage was a society of procreation.

Desire fascinates: *fascinus* was the Roman word for phallus. It is always represented in erection, as opposed to the *mensula* (the penis) in a state of flaccidity. In Rome, a man is in an erect state. The state of flaccidity was a distressing obsession. His horror of *mensula* leads him to the search for power, a search that perhaps characterizes man. Ejaculation is a voluptuous loss, but the loss of arousal, and therefore erection, is something that worries the man at all times Aristotle defines the male sex what increases and decreases in volume: metamorphosis.

Men are perhaps afraid of women, and we can hypothesize several reasons. In the apocryphal Old Testament, the only being who challenged God head-on was Lilith, by pronouncing His name. Considered demonic, she is credited with visiting the dreams of young people and using the semen of her nocturnal pollution to conceive children. Then Eve, with the tree of knowledge, tempted Adam to sin. In Greek mythology, Pandora lifted the lid of the jar, allowing evils to be poured out on men.

Since Tiresias (Grimal, 1951), who was a woman before being a man, we know that out of ten parts of pleasure, nine correspond to women, and only one to men. For revealing this knowledge, Zeus punished him by transforming him into a serpent. Attributing to women an insatiable capacity for pleasure makes men fearful. The *fascinus* disappears in the vulva and comes out *mensula*, that is, flaccid. The man perhaps fears revenge for failing to satisfy the woman fully.

Perhaps, like Perseus before the Medusa, every man approaches the woman fearfully, with a protective shield. He fears, like anyone who approaches the Medusa, being paralyzed. The woman gives life, and every human being comes from the womb of a woman. But at the same time death is embodied in mythology by the figure of three women: the Grim Reapers. Between unbridled sexuality and death, we find the figure of the praying mantis, which kills her partner after intercourse. The man may be afraid of the woman because he thinks that she may be envious of his penis—a theory long disseminated by orthodox psychoanalysis, but which seems to me the result of a male theorizing. To the representation of the all-powerful woman, the man responds with the desire for domination, as a representation created to evacuate his fear.

If for Freud the woman was the dark continent, bearer of an enigma like the Sphinx of Thebes, Leticia Glocer-Fiorini (2015) emphasizes that in reality the dark continent and the enigma is not the woman but the Other, all other, beyond her gender, which by its condition of otherness generates a disturbing question. It is as disturbing as the unconscious itself, unknowable through reflection. The foundational decentralization in relation to the other and to his irreducible alienation. But at the same time, regarding the decentralization itself, by putting the axis not so much in consciousness, but in the unconscious. Both decentralizations are the main sources of concern for every human being, even without prejudging their anatomical condition, gender, or the forms that their sexualities may take. The originality of psychoanalysis consists in the privileged relationship that ties its object of study, that is, the unconscious, to the sexual.

Movements for sexual liberation, the empowerment of women, have an indisputable social value. The possibility of living one's sexuality freely, as long as it does not constitute a crime, is an advance in the notion not only of sexual freedom, but of human freedom. It is no accident if authoritarian regimes stifle sexual liberation. A sad example has been the persecution of homosexuals by the Nazis or, even without going so far, during the military regime in Argentina (1976–1982).

But it is advisable not to deceive ourselves: although sexual freedom is a liberating advance of the human condition, it does not eliminate the notion of conflict associated with sexuality. There is no such thing as a fully happy sexuality. The conscious Self is not king. Unlike Louis XIV, who said, "I am the state," the Self cannot affirm that psychic life is the Self. The other psychic instances, the impulsive pole of it and the categorical mandates of the superego intervene together. Whatever form human sexuality takes, it is always a psycho-sexuality, and as such it is not without conflicts between instances.

Psychoanalysis is not sexology but, rather, archaeology, a setting in history. Sexual life, its most intimate part, is not the result of acquired knowledge: it is a particular alchemy that defines us from our earliest years. Sexuality is not chosen on the shelf of a supermarket: sexuality defines us more than we choose it. Returning to the initial question of this debate, I do not think that masculinities are in check. If something related to a distorted form of masculinity is in check, it is chauvinism, a distorting mirror of it.

In a traditionally hetero-patriarchal society the condition of man gave a certain place of certainty, whereras today masculinity is in constant re-definition, shaking the caricature of the masculine, removing the mask of superhero, putting the masculine on a par with the feminine—a masculinity that is nourished by femininity, one's own and others', and that is not violent with the feminine. The risk would be that the man projects into the woman his own rejected femininity, sometimes reaching an unusual violence, an extreme way of denying himself and all bisexuality present in every human being.

I don't think feminist and LGBTQ+ movements put masculinities in check. They question the patriarchal hierarchy; they fight for equal civic rights, which is not the same thing. Times have changed; it is likely that the unconscious of men will take time to notice. Meanwhile, a woman is murdered every 36 hours in Argentina—and the situation is similar in many other countries. There is urgency in deconstructing a masculinity confused with the hetero-patriarchal chauvinism hierarchy.

References

Deleuze, G., & Guattari, F. (1976). *Rhizome*. Paris: Ed. de Minuit.

Derrida, J. (1967). *L'écriture et la difference*. Paris: Seuil.

Glocer-Fiorini, L. (2015). *La diferencia sexual en debate*. Buenos Aires: Lugar Editorial.

Grimal, P. (1951). *Dictionnaire de la mythologie grecque et romaine*. Paris: PUF.

Lacan, J. (1975). *Le séminaire, Livre XX. Encore*. Paris: Éditions du Seuil,

Morin, E. (1914). *Introduction à la pensée complexe*. Paris: Points.

Quignard, P. (1994). *Le sexe et l'effroi*. Paris: Gallimard,

Volnovich, J. C., & Rodulfo, R. (1997). Prologue [to Spanish edition]. In: J. Benjamin, *Like Subjects, Love Objects, Essays on Recognition and Sexual Difference*. Spanish edition, Buenos Aires: Paidós; original English edition, New Haven, CT: Yale University Press, 1995.

12 The tattoo and the shield of Perseus*

The term "tattoo" finds its origin in the islands of Polynesia, and reveals the link between tattooing and animistic thinking attributed to societies misnamed "primitive." In these islands, everything that existed on earth was animated by the *Atuás*, that is, the spirits. Drawing (*ta* = drawing) the spirit on the body by means of a *ta-atuás* allowed the person to benefit from the favors of that spirit, or to protect oneself from its punishments. For the primitive inhabitants of Tahiti, the tattoo was a skin reflection of a mode of social functioning.

In the history of tattooing, we find that it is not only mythical sailors who made use of it. Although there is no reliable evidence, it is legitimate to assume that the tattoo appeared with *Homo sapiens* 50,000 years ago, in prehistory and at the time of the appearance of graphics on the walls of caves. The tattoo may have existed since people had begun writing. It is important to underline the initial place of the body as a sign in the societies of *H. sapiens* in Europe (Vialou, 1998). We found tangible evidence of tattooing in Egypt, on mummies. For example, and as an anecdotal value, the priestess Hathour Amounet, who was a royal concubine (2160 BC), had tattoos on her left shoulder, on her belly, in the subpubic region, and on the inner thighs. Initially abstract, tattoos became figurative in the era of the New Empire. Often figurations of the God Bes, reserved for women, are interpreted by Egyptologists in terms of erogeneity and reinforcement of the power of female seduction. The tattoo is, then, in this distant origin linked to Eros. The three great monotheistic religions would later condemn all practices of ornamentation and voluntary modification of the image of the body, trying to repress all erogenous significance. The tattoo became a sign of divine power, punishment, and, at the same time, protection, as with God and Cain: "God put a sign on Cain so that whoever finds him does not kill him." If God can tattoo the sinner, it is forbidden

* A first version of this text was published in the *Journal of the Argentine Association of Psychology and Group Psychotherapy*, Vol. 23, No. 2, 2000, Buenos Aires; and in the *Revue Adolescence*, Vol. 21, No. 3, 2003, Paris.

DOI: 10.4324/9781032647791-15

for man to tattoo himself. In *Leviticus, 19*: 28 we find: "They will not make incisions in your skin and will not imprint figures on it." The icons are be extra-corporeal and reserved for divine images.

We owe the English navigator James Cook the renewed interest in tattooing in the eighteenth century. The meticulous cartographer describes the practice of tattooing in the Polynesian islands and transcribes for the first time into English the term "Tattoo", as the natives called it. The tattoo was to become fashionable, and the greatest Polynesian tattoo artists came to Europe. Edward VII, George V and George VI of England, Frederick of Prussia, Count Tolstoy, Tsar Nicholas, and many others would experience such art. However, the concept of the tattoo was degraded in Europe in the nineteenth century, to the extent that the great criminologists, such as Lombroso, considered it a specific anatomical–legal characteristic of the criminal. It was not until the 1930s that Locard said that the mere fact of a tattoo does not allow concuding that it applies to a special category of men (Tenenhaus, 1993).

When talking about tattooing in history, one cannot ignore the ignominious use that the Nazis made of it in concentration camps, with the tattoo of numbers, euphemistically called "identification," actually of de-subjectivation of prisoners. But this is not, in a strict sense, a tattoo: it is an imposed mark, an affront against humanity via a number that indicated the attempted extermination of a community—a mark of death, no longer linked to Eros, as in early times, but to Thanatos.

In our contemporary societies, the voluntary act of tattooing is an individual gesture and is, in that sense, a private act: however, the trace on the skin, its graphics, is read in public and frequently shows belonging to a given group, depending on age, culture, or other parameters.

In my clinical presentation I will therefore limit myself to voluntary tattoos and their unconscious basis. From a psychodynamic perspective, and beyond the common cultural values that are usually displayed in the choice of tattoos, I think it is important to underline the heterogeneous character of tattoos from a metapsychological point of view, their polysemic character. Beyond the current fashion among adolescents to get tattoos, I will not make a sociological study of them, but a psychodynamic proposal.

In the manner of the image of a dream, the tattoo is, above all, the graphic expression of a psychic production of the subject. The voluntary tattoo becomes an act of language halfway between a writing that approaches the hieroglyph, with its symbolisms, and discursive orality. As a substitutive representation, the image printed on the skin acquires the metonymic value of the internal world, but not necessarily its metaphorical value.

In the short story "The Illustrated Man," the character imagined by Ray Bradbury (1955) has his entire body tattooed: there is nowhere, on his body, that is free of tattoos. At night, when the character falls asleep, each tattoo becomes animated, takes on a life of its own, and gives rise to a story: "Each illustration is a story. If you look at them for a few minutes, they will tell you a story. If you look at them for three hours, the narratives will be thirty or forty, and you will hear voices, and thoughts. It's all here in my skin; just look." The observer came to look at 18 tattoos that gave rise to 18 stories. But if you heard those same voices, … the narratives could be endless…. thousand and one stories.

Nicolás and his tattoos

I now present Nicolás, my patient, and his story, in the framework of his analysis, in which I stress what concerns his tattoos and their metapsychological value.

At the time of the consultation, Nicolás was 17 years old. He was referred to me as a case of major depression: isolated, confined to a room in his house in an attitude of at once passive and narcissistic withdrawal, without contacts with other adolescents except those offered by school—a school that, despite his state, he manages to attend. The parents are extremely concerned about their eldest son, whom they describe as a boy who had always been quiet during his childhood, obedient, rather taciturn. At the time of the consultation, he does not show interest in any social activity, maintaining, as his only interest, music and his long guitar solos. He sleeps a lot, doesn't play sports, doesn't go out with friends and doesn't study. However, his good intellectual capacity has allowed him to spend the year in a private school, where he starts the last year of high school. The only outings he manages are to go with his father to the soccer stadium of his favorite team, Boca, where they attend regularly, as they have a season ticket. The family moved from Buenos Aires to Mar del Plata, a city in the interior of Argentina, a few years earlier, when Nicolás was 8 years old. The parents are merchants and share the opening hours of the family business. Beyond the indication of the colleague who referred him to me for therapy, the father welcomes the proposal, because he clarifies that, having had an analysis himself a few years earlier, he is able to verify the benefits it brought him. Nicolás had a history of hypothyroidism, so he was medicated from the age of 13. The consultation comes shortly after one of his 16-year-old friends made a suicide attempt, which had worried the whole family.

Nicolás is an introverted teenager, shy, smooth, who does not let out his words or his light brown hair, which is cut extremely short. He has a dull, languid look; his stature seems shorter than average because of the attitude of his slumped shoulders. The tone of his voice is monotonous, but I wouldn't say gray. Some colors appear in the first meeting. He is initially a little skeptical about the interview, but at the same time curious about the proposal to say everything that goes through his head and, in particular, that whatever is said is part of professional confidentiality, from which even his parents and a younger brother are excluded. He was not used to confidentiality: in the name of love and transparency of family relationships, thoughts had to be debated in the family group, making it difficult to preserve intimacy. The family was where action and violence had predominated as a form of exchange.

An adolescent, as is well known, faces several duels that require a process of elaboration of loss, typical of this age, requiring important psychic work. The adolescent must mourn his parents of childhood and the omnipotence he conferred on them, losing, together with their omnipotence, the protection against death. He must mourn his infant body that kept him protected from the impulsive drives that arises with violence at puberty. By reactivation and re-issue of the oedipal problematic he confronts the mourning of his own omnipotence, the mourning of androgynous bisexuality and symbolic castration. It is no small feat. How many adults do we know who have never made it? Among the multiple ways offered to the adolescent, from the preferable symbolic elaboration to the pathological solution such as mania, psychopathy, the tendency to the passage to the act, etc., Nicolas had unconsciously found the depressive "solution." It was the expression of struggle in the face of the emergence of a threatening and chaotic inner world. The fragility of his internal objects, Nicolás's representational emptiness, put him on the edge of the abyss where he could fall at any moment. His immobility was the way he had found to try to stop the vertigo to which he felt compelled.

With the variable regularity that characterizes adolescents, Nicolás invests in his therapy and the possibility of talking about himself. In a short time, he manages to leave his cystic room and open up to the world. Football and music will be the two pillars that will allow him to leave his long soliloquy with less fear. He returns to the sport and starts playing indoor football with friends. They organize a team, and at the end of the year participate in a tournament promoted by a commercial brand, the team winning a graduation holiday. This idea pleases him doubly. Having already organized and paid for his graduate trip to Bariloche, the prize obtained will allow him to travel again the following year, becoming a second graduate holiday, a possibility that allowed him to enjoy the fantasy of graduating a second time, thus delaying the passage of time. The recurring theme of the therapy had been his anguish in the face of the black hole that opened up after finishing high school. The prospects were immense: they opened up, for him, not so much an opening choice but a fall into a world, he said, "that he could be crushed by"—an expression that revealed both his real perception of the risks of the contemporary world and his renewed castration anxiety. He quickly manages to get two friends with whom he would share outings, conversation, and his passion for music throughout the year. He attends rock recitals, and goes to punk-rock, heavy-metal groups, and groups with funnier lyrics: protest—he tells me. He also tells me that in his childhood he suffered a lot because he went unnoticed in the group: "When I was a kid there were two groups at school, one that studied and another that played sports. I was neither in one nor the other. In class it was like I wasn't there." He clarifies to me that he likes to be looked at, to be taken into account.

After a long journey Nicolás decided to study journalism, a choice that arose from his desire to go to study in Buenos Aires, a project that would allow him to simultaneously return to his grandparents' house, where he had lived until he was 8 years old. Nicolas was anxious about separating from his friends, who represented his longed-for group of belonging. One of them planned to go with his parents to live in Spain, another would stay in Mar del Plata, and he would go to Buenos Aires. Because of a lack of time, I cannot discuss all the nuances of a psychotherapy that proved extremely rich. I will talk only about the metapsychological function that his tattoo projects acquired. Faced with the anguish of separation, the three friends decided that they would get the same tattoo, of symbols representing rock groups and the logo of another punk rock group. He tells me about the place where tattooing is practiced and the technique used. And he adds that a third picture will probably be made. I ask him whether he needs the agreement of his parents, and he replies that in any case the following week he turns 18, and that he will be able to make the decision alone. That is to say that he announces to me that his body belongs to him and that he has the freedom to mark it, and, although he does not formulate it in this way, it is implicit in his speech that he even possesses the power to destroy it. He tells me that he will first do two tattoos, in relation to rock bands, leaving a third, with the image of a snake, for later, because the mother requires him first to pass mathematics, a subject that he had been failing since 4th year—a situation that had been hidden from the father. In that same session he brings the following story of a dream: "he looks in the mirror and has his entire torso and chest tattooed, from the waist up." He tells me that he liked that image, that it was a dream that brought him tranquility. Instead, another dream from the same night is disturbing to him: "He sees himself in the mirror with a beard and doesn't like it." It was not so much their imaginary associations that we take up, as the affective pendulum movement lived in both dreams: the serene tranquility of the former in opposition to the pronounced anguish of the latter.

The importance of the function of the mirror in relation to castration anxiety in the two dreams is well known. Having the whole chest and torso tattooed "from the waist up" is the full graphic image that leaves no empty spaces, that leaves no holes. In the obliteration of the gaze on what would pass below the waist, Nicolás avoids confrontation with castration anxiety. The tranquility of the first dream expresses denial of this anxiety. In the dream of the beard, on the other hand, his anguish of growing up clearly appears, of assimilating the changes in his body and in his sexuality, expressed by the visualization of the secondary sexual characteristics of the appearance of the beard.

Regarding tattoos—both those in the dream and those that he plans to have done— Nicolás tells me: "I like my body to change." Thus, it is he who produces the changes in his body, in the illusion of dominating them, not the body that changes in spite of him. A third dream from another session completes the cycle: "He's going to play football, and they were about to get him a third tattoo, it was a snake. It was his mathematics teacher and a friend of his father who were going to do it." There appears, in this last dream, a clear feeling of anguish in relation to castration. The mathematics teacher, a persecutory figure, even more so to the extent that he shared with Nicolás's mother the exclusion of the father from the information about the exam he has yet to pass, associated with the father to leave an indelible mark on his body. That the image chosen was a snake is not accidental, given its highly evocative power of the denial of castration, whose top is represented by the head of the Medusa from which multiple snakes emanate and whose phallic value was highlighted by Freud (1940 [1922], p. 270) in his article on the Gorgon. The image was a clear exponent of his castration anxiety, whose agent in the dream was represented by a surrogate father figure, his mathematics teacher, in complicity with the mother. Oedipal anguish of a compromise between the oedipal desire to exclude the father, given the connivance of the same with the mathematics teacher, and the persecutory presence of the father through said teacher. The chosen tattoo both causes a wound and simultaneously leaves an indelible mark in the service of the denial of loss.

We can say that, generally, the impulsive excitement is in search of representations. When psychic representations fail, the inscription of a graphic representation on the skin can serve a substitute function for representation—halfway between psychic representation and external object, in-between, not totally on the outside, but not on the inside. It fulfills a symbolic but not necessarily metaphorical function.

"In dreams we do not feel horror because we are oppressed by a sphinx, we dream a sphinx to explain the horror we feel," says Borges (1974). The psychic apparatus does not admit that affection is left floating. The affectionate representative of the drive is Pirandellian, as in *Six Characters in Search of an Author* (1921): affection seeks a representation where it can anchor, otherwise it is the overflowing emergency of anguish. The tattoo snake absorbs the castration anxiety that cannot be contained by a metabolizable psychic elaboration of it. The image of the tattoo becomes the representation of the commitment of castration anxiety and its denial.

In our patient Nicolás, the representative capacity of the primary process that is expressed through sleep was overwhelmed by homosexual drives and castration anxiety. The representative potentiality of sleep was exceeded in its capacity to symbolize the conflicts of psychic bisexuality. The tattoo, as a support of a psychic projection in his own body, allows him to live the representation as outside himself and, simultaneously, in his own body—an apparent exteriority that makes it more tolerable. It is an outside of the psyche in its corporeal ego, an externalized interiority, but not lost in the limitless external world, but contained by a wrapper that functions as an interface between the internal and external worlds. Continence of his psyche is also sought through the sound envelope of rock music. The tattoo became a compromise between the impossibility of containing the conflicts within his psychic life proper to metaphorizable thought, and an expulsion outside oneself, in a non-recognition of the fantastic production as one's own. It is a first attempt to elaborate a failing psychic economy and from which the body pays its tribute—the tattoo as a pictogram, as an expression of original thought, of which Piera Aulagnier (1975) spoke, the tattoo as a figuration of an unthinkable halfway to a thinkable in order to become sayable. The skin in its condition of psychic wrapping, of a skin-ego (Anzieu, 1985. 1987), of a border between the external world and the internal world, contains in the inscription of the tattoo the re-presentation of fragile object relations. It allows a lessening of the anguish, whether of castration, loss of the object, or fragmentation. In his search for containment of his anguish, Nicolás found the sound wrapping of rock music, reinforced by the tattoos represented by the different rock groups: icons, simultaneously, of an initiatory rite, of belonging to a group identity, and an attempt to elaborate their psychic bisexuality and the ties of homosexual content so frequent at that time of life. To the incessant struggle against his primary depression was added the mourning of the separation from his friends. Faced with the blurred contours of the negativity of the shadow of the lost object, Nicolás preferred the positive sharpness (as they say about a photograph) of the image of tattoos inscribing itself on the surface of his body—in-between, between the perforated interior that let the internal object escape and an exterior that sucked it into the void.

The indelible mark of the tattoo as a certainty of no change in the face of the transformations operating in the body independently of itself is an anchor point of a certain timelessness. "To have as embedded in the body a still time" (Pelento, 1998) that is not subject to the avatars of the unconscious desire of the subject or to the uncertainties of the desire of the Other and of the ungraspable external world. Thus, the tattoo can represent a time in parentheses, which, like an immobile time, provides the illusion of a time stopped, allowing the body not to suffer the inexorable avatars of chronological time.

If the skin partially fails in its condition as a mirror that allows it to recognize and measure the outside, to clothe it sufficiently, and to see itself at the same time investing its own image, it nevertheless offers a surface of inscription to the unconscious production of the subject. To the chaos of the unrepresentable of their own bodily transformations, the tattoo proposes to the adolescent a trace not yet represented, but representable and organizing of senses.

Does the adolescent, deep down, get tattooed to feel looked at, or to refract the gaze of the other? The question is not superfluous and the answer is less obvious than it seems at first glance. A quick passage through mythology will allow me to clarify, I hope, what I mean.

Perseus, in order to prevent the advances of the tyrant Polydectes on his mother Danae, undertakes to obtain for him the head of Medusa (Grimal, 1976). Medusa, I may recall, is one of the three Gorgons. Her head is surrounded by snakes; she had bronze hands and golden wings that allowed her to fly. Her tongue was violently sticking out, above a bearded chin. She was frightening, with her penetrating and resplendent gaze that turned anyone who looked at her into stone. Perseus manages to behead her, thanks to his courage, and also thanks to the help of Hermes and Athena, who provide him with winged sandals, a sword, and a shield. To avoid looking at her, Perseus uses his polished bronze shield: this, like a mirror, reflects the gaze of the Medusa. With this trick the Medusa is petrified with the reflection of her own gaze. Avoiding the paralyzing gaze of the Medusa, Perseus manages to decapitate her.

For Francis Pasche (1971), the psychic apparatus should be able to benefit from a shield form, like that of Perseus. This psychic shield would have two main functions: (1) as a protective wrapping that aids in resisting external forces and, in particular, tin putting a limit on the feared aspect of the phallic mother (Medusa) and therefore autonomy. (2) A mirror that allows recognition and evaluation of the outside, but also sufficient investment in it, which saves the paroxysm of anguish that triggers the mutual confrontation of the impulses of life and death in the presence of the object vacuum.

Freud, in his article on Medusa's head, points out that the horror produced by the Medusa makes it equivalent to beheading with castrating. The jellyfish terror is, then, a castration anxiety related to the sight of something. And Freud attributes this something to the effect on the child of the observation of the differences between the sexes. It is remarkable, Freud points out, how the snakes on Medusa's head, despite being horrible in themselves, mitigate the horror, as the multiplicity of phallic symbols attenuates the castration anxiety.

Returning to Nicolás, it seemed to me that the tattoo of the serpent, metonymic representative of the phallus, means the same thing that Freud maintained in that article: I am not afraid of you, I challenge you, I have the phallus. In other words, the tattoo, made to be seen, acquires thea fetishistic value of a denial of castration, like a veil that allows it to both show and to hide, as if it wanted to say: "when you look at my tattoo, you do not see the rest of my body."

We find, in Nicolás's tattoo, an aspect of protective psychic shield of which F. Pasche spoke. Attracting the gaze of others to the tattoo in order to divert it from the rest of your body is one of the functions of tattooing in the adolescent—as if the sex difference were too distressing to be seen from the front, having to go through an oblique look, responding to both the prohibition of looking back (Orpheus) and the prohibition of looking straight ahead (Medusa).

They are the representatives of psychic contents that express the struggle for psychic survival. The tattoo and its representational value to Nicolás was an attempt to skirt the representational void to which he feared being aspired and to protect his bodily self from falling into it, reinforcing a system of hesitant repression.

Finally, I will say that adolescence has a traumatogenic potential in the Freudian sense of the term, that is, the risk that the subject experiences by seeing his capacity for elaboration and libidinal reorganization over-whelmed by the task that adolescence requires. In this sense, the process of adolescence implies a demand for psychic work in order to contain, give meaning to, and organize the transformations that affect adolescence and that occur in spite of it. Where the adolescent is passivated in the face of a change that he suffers and does not dominate, it is gener-ated by the re-issue of his Oedipus complex, but also by the process of separation–individuation and the confrontation with the limitless space of the extra-familiar. It is the staging, but also the attempt to put in the sense of an unspeakable affection. Sometimes intra-psychic representations are scarce to prefigure this change, and the tattoo is an attempt to offer on the surface of the body the anchor to a representation of a wandering affection that tears him apart as not yet tellable.

References

Anzieu, D. (1985). *Le moi-peau*. Paris: Dunod.

Anzieu, D. (1987). Les signifiants formels et le moi-peau. In: *Les enveloppes psy-chiques*, Paris: Dunod.

Aulagnier, P. (1975). *La violence de l'interprétation. Du pictogramme à l'énoncé*. Paris: PUF.

Borges, J. L. (1974). El hacedor. In: *Obras Completas*. Buenos Aires: Emecé.

Bradbury, R. (1955). *El hombre ilustrado* [The illustrated man]. Buenos Aires: Mino-tauro, 1998.

Freud, S. (1940 [1922]). Medusa's head. In: *Standard Edition, Vol. 18*. London: Hog-arth Press.

Grimal, P. (1976). *Dictionnaire de la mythologie grecque et romaine*. Paris: PUF.

Pasche, F. (1971). Le bouclier de Persée ou psychose et réalité. *Revue Française de Psychanalyse, 35* (5–6).

Pelento, M. L. (1998). Los tatuajes como marcas. *Revista de Psicoanálisis, Buenos Aires, 56* (2).

Pirandello, L. (1921). *Sei personaggi in cerca d'autore* [Six characters in search of an author]. Milan: Tascabili, 1993.

Tenenhaus, H. (1993). *Le tatouage à l'adolescence*. Paris: Bayard.

Vialou, D. (1998). Sexualité et art préhistoriques. In F. Sacco (Ed.), *Le propre de l'homme*. Lausanne: Delauchaux et Niestlé.

13 William, did you say, "Much ado about nothing"?

Anatomy is no longer destiny, and sexual identities do not depend on any aesthetic. The notion of gender has de-reified the biological, and, after a long period of gender binarism, *queer* theory questions it and postulates multiplicity beyond the dichotomy of genders. The intersexuality and intergender that plead against binarism and in favor of a flexible sexuality not assigned from birth question psychoanalysis and create a need for us to deconstruct and reformulate several of our paradigms. In psychoanalysis it is nearly impossible to speak of a woman or a man, not only because we need to use the plural, but most of all because it is impossible to consider this from an a-historical or a-cultural perspective. No naturalistic essentialism of woman or man is able to transcend the symbolic construction of its era. Therefore, speaking about women and creativity is a difficult challenge in terms of psychoanalysis. I will therefore allow myself a detour, something like a tangential look; we know that a frontal gaze may "medusa" more than one of us, and looking back may turn us into a statue of salt.

It is well known that the anatomic difference between the sexes (Freud, 1925b) initially poses questions for girls and boys ... and probably for all adults, for the rest of their lives. The drive to know or epistemophilia is rooted in this questioning. In his phallocentric theory, Freud postulates, in boys, castration anxiety and in girls penis envy as prototypes of the decline of the Oedipus complex (Freud, 1924). The girl thinks, at first, that it will grow, and, disillusioned because her mother did not give it to her, she turns toward her father, without better results. She finally leaves her Oedipus behind via the penis–child equation. Obviously, we remain in the dark regarding the fate of women who have not had at least one child and do not know whether those who have had more than one have resolved their Oedipus faster, or whether they have had several children because they were unable to resolve it. ... Freud considers only one libido, which is essentially masculine, although there is no difference between the sexes in the unconscious, and in this sense human sexuality could never be complementary.

Little is said of the boy's envy of the girl, although several eminent authors have described something that those of us who have a clinical

DOI: 10.4324/9781032647791-16

practice with children have been able to confirm, which is boys' envy of girls. Boys want to have breasts or to get pregnant, adhering later to the cloaca theory. As Lucile Durrmeyer (1999) points out, this envy is joined by another that boys may have: envy of the "ideal penis," meaning one that could always be erect (the Roman *fascinus*) or even make it longer, as so well described in Louis Pergaud's *Guerre des Boutons* [War of the Buttons] in which the boys compete with each other to see who can piss furthest. In recent years, multiple spam emails arrive via the internet promising their potential and unwitting clients the sexual panacea of lengthening their penis.

We could also mention men's envy of women's capacity for sexual pleasure as revealed by Tiresias, the memorable blind man who had been a woman before being a man and attributed nine parts of pleasure in ten to women and only one to men (Tesone, 2006).

Jessica Benjamin (1995) postulates an over-inclusive conception of the genders: the girl or boy wishes to be and have everything, in a narcissistic omnipotence that no adult abandons completely.

Freud underscored the double possibilities of identification in every individual, from which psychic bisexuality results. Much was said about gender identity as if it were something stable, attained once and for all, whereas it seems to me that a precipitate of both genders often remains which removes it far from the fixedness of an immobile identity, thereby allowing subjectivation that is much richer in complexity and movements inside the psyche. The contemporary ego is a fragmented and many-faceted ego, an experience unrelated to psychotic fragmentation but, rather to different facets of the ego.

The literary production of Pessoa and his multiple heteronyms that converse with each other, have diverse styles, fight over literary issues and even have different dates and places of birth is a good example of this potential richness that made Pessoa the greatest Portuguese poet of our time.

What is the impact of the anatomical difference between the sexes on human beings from the phantasmatic and symbolic perspective? Much has been said and much has been negated. Some theories function as veils and thereby acquire value as fetishes. When Shakespeare wrote his play, *Much Ado About Nothing* in 1600, in the form of a comedy, a Renaissance conception of women was placed in tension. His text distills subtle irony regarding prejudices about women and men in his time. On the lips of Beatrice, he sets incisive and provocative dialogue in a duel between equals with Benedick, unusual for his era; they mutually deny love. but finally become spouses. Through Hero, the daughter of Leonato, all of men's fears concerning women's infidelity appear, as well as the seal of disapproval reserved for women if they are not virgins when they marry. We may assume that this play is a satire on the condition of women and that it was not worth making such "ado" about Hero's allegedly missing virginity or her false infidelity. However, "nothing" in Elizabethan slang means vagina. Therefore, "nothing" was intended to mean that women had nothing (no-thing) between their legs. I would like to discuss this term *nothing* in greater detail.

The slip from the penis to the phallus proposed by Lacan (this concept is complex and requires further development) enabled at least a desacralization of anatomy, but still positions both genders in relation to the phallic order. "The male position is ruled by having and the feminine position is based on lack in being. For men it is a question of having the phallus in order to be in a position to give it, and for women not to have it in order to be able to desire it" (Chaboudez, 1994, p. 27). Tension is produced between being and having, but the order still turns upon the phallus, the only symbol of desire for both sexes, although Lacan also spoke of gender, departing from biological binarism, when in his famous formulation about sexuation Lacan (1972–1973, p. 67), he spoke about the feminine position and the masculine position. He cites the mystics to exemplify this: Saint John of the Cross occupying a feminine position in his poems. However, he does not discard binarism, although he does drop the idea of complementarity between the sexes. Leticia Glocer (Glocer-Fiorini, 2001) proposes understanding the feminine position with the help of Edgar Morin's (2007) notion of complex thought, which consists in considering two propositions recognized as being true, but that seem to exclude each other mutually as two faces of a complex truth in a relation of interdependence. This author reminds us that since the origins of psychoanalysis, the feminine has appeared to be an obstacle to any hope of coherence and integration of the theory.

In this point of view, Freud's dark continent would be an expression of the unexplored and the enigmatic, but also of complexity exceeding the phallic register.

In relation to the phallic order, is there nothing in the sense of a void … or does nothing acquire existence? The invisibility of female sex organs has often been compared to nothing, to negativity, to the point that debates about whether girls had a notion of the existence of their vagina before or after puberty was interminable. A famous controversy was in 1926 raised by Karen Horney (1967), when she questioned Freud's hypothesis: unlike him, she stated that this alleged ignorance of the vagina was a product of repression (Horney, 1967).

Before continuing with this representation of the female sex, I will take a detour through the notion of nothing in Heidegger. What is nothing? Asks the philosopher in his text, *what is metaphysics?* (Heidegger, 2000). Any metaphysical question, he explains, may only be formulated in such a way "that the person who asks—as such—is also included in the question, that is to say, is also questioned in it" (p. 94). Why does Heidegger ask about nothing? Precisely because science rejects nothing and discards it, because it is nothing. For science, nothing is nothing more than a reason for horror and a phantasmagoria, he deduces. Boys and girls behave just the same way, as if they were investigators perturbed by their object of study. If thinking is always thinking about something, then thinking about nothing would essentially be a logical contradiction. "Would there only be nothing because there is a no? Does nothingness represent the no and negativity and therefore negation? Or is it the other way around? Is there negation and the no because there is nothing?" (p. 95). A methodological inversion that subverts reasoning and thinking about nothingness and negation. However, if "come what may, nothingness must be questioned, then previously it has to have been given." (p. 95). In French, nothingness is *"le néant,"* which is to say "non-entity."

In consequence, if nothingness is not considered, then we can only believe in the existence of an entity. When we leave behind the existence of entity and come close to the nothingness that is non-entity, this generates anxiety: "Anxiety reveals nothingness," states Heidegger (2000, p. 3). Anxiety "leaves us without words." Since entity completely escapes us, this would be the way nothingness questions us. In the face of nothingness, "all pretense of saying that something 'is' falls silent" (p. 104).

The German philosopher maintains that nothingness does not attract but, due to its essence, repels. How can we help thinking about the boy's reaction, but also the girl's, to castration anxiety when they confront the invisibility of the female sex? *"Dasein"* [being there] means being immersed in nothingness. Without the originary manifest quality of nothingness, there would be no being-oneself or any freedom at all. In this sense, "nothingness is not the concept opposite to entity but pertains originarily to being itself" (Heidegger, 2000, p. 106). For psychoanalysis, it is not a matter of indifference to follow the development of his thought when he states that nothingness is the origin of negation, and not vice versa. However, negation is not the only component of entity's desisting supremacy; bitterness is also produced "in deprivation and in renouncement" (p. 107).

Paraphrasing Jessica Benjamin (1995), we could say that giving up the narcissism of being and having everything is not a simple thing for human beings or something that can be entirely resolved.

Originary anxiety, related to nothingness, as Heidegger states, may awaken at any moment in the *Dasein*. He quotes Hegel when he considers pure being and pure nothingness to be the same, that is to say, being and nothingness mutually pertaining to each other.

Therefore, we propose that the discovery of the difference between the sexes involves including nothingness in the two sexes as a logical necessity. Historically, male bias pushed nothingness into the female sex with the facilitation of the non-visibility of the woman's sex, folded inward. The female sex came to represent nothingness as a projection of a masculine cultural dominance that was too preoccupied with projecting into women lack, emptiness, nothingness, and the negative of "having" the phallus venerated by all cultures as a symbol of fertility.

Plutarch (cited by Quignard, 1994, p. 98) writes that the ithyphallic amulet attracts the gaze of the fascinated—hence the incredible arsenal of amulets, burlesque dwarves, in gold, ivory, stone, bronze, all in priapic form, essential in archeological explorations.

Mariam Alizade (1992) praises nothingness and emphasizes nothingness in women, both in their biological dimension and in the phantasms based on this biology. She states that "the concept of nothingness in psychoanalysis is on the opposite side of the street from the phallus" (p. 27).

Her position is close to Heidegger's, given that he maintains that this is "a nothingness that has a name. There is positivity and participation in nothingness. Nothingness exists. The second way to consider nothingness places it beside the impossible, the unnamable, the unrepresentable and the unthinkable" (Alizade, 1992, p. 32).

However, for Alizade, this nothingness is a productive and fertile nothingness, even though the human subject tries to avoid the "encounter or contact with these effects of nothingness by means of excessive discrimination, fixedness of oppositions and certainty of concepts" (Alizade, 1992, p. 45).

In reality, it is nothingness that persists and finds the subject, evoking the archaic, the uncanny, and the demonic, leaving an invisible, mute trail. She adds the "nothingy" order to the phallic order. It is characterized primarily by the installation of a knowledge of lack, a knowledge supported beyond anxiety. This order constantly touches on the real, where the psychic uproar of the phallic is. All phallic power allows avoidance of confrontation with lack and finitude. It is on the woman's body that the horror of the truth materializes, "the *horror feminae*, designated an enigma" (Alizade, 1992, p. 56). Both mystery and death are condensed in the woman's body. Having the phallus facilitates projection of the representation of absence. As extreme solutions to the anxiety aroused by nothingness, the fetish object sutures the place of lack, and erotomania fills lack with certainty of the object's love. When disavowal seizes the throne, the pleasure ego disavows the traumatizing perception. In this sense, phallic value acquires the power of reassurance to ward off anxiety of lack in both sexes.

Behind the phallic order lies hidden a narcissistic omnipotence that conceals "a deeper, subjacent and silent order" (Alizade, 1992, p. 65), where Eros and Thanatos are intimately fused and in which incompleteness is conceived as circulating in a creative way. What is important for Alizade—and I concur—is that nothingness should not be expelled, both sexes accepting that nothingness concerns them equally, that this nothingness includes the mystery of life and death for both sexes in the same measure.

It is no coincidence that the outset of life is represented as the figure of a woman, as creating, and the end of life as one of the Fates. Gustave Courbet's "The Origin of the World", which represents the vulva as a painting, probably provoked questions for Lacan; he nonetheless in some way concealed it by not making it public—although he was its owner—and by keeping it in his country house. After his death, as payment of death taxes, it was turned over to the *Musée d'Orsay*, where it continues to provoke questions in its numerous viewers.

The world, things, the other, and each part of the other have no other presence "than the painting that is made out of them," in the words of Corinne Enaudeau (1998), who adds, "All that is authentic is only a substitute, image or word" (p. 54). Courbet's image, like a mirror, duplicates the representation of the female sex. But the image does not judge: it illustrates the thing.

In his article "Negation," Freud (1925) states that judgment of attribution precedes judgment of existence: "The function of judgment is concerned in the main with two sorts of decisions. It affirms or disaffirms the possession by a thing of a particular attribute; and it asserts or disputes that a presentation has an existence in reality" (p. 236).

It is inherent to thought to rise above pure activity of representation, but there is no thought that is not influenced by perception, and, conversely, perception is not a purely passive process. In the seventeenth century, Caravaggio (cited by Quignard, 1994, p. 23) said that every painting is a Medusa's head. Terror may be defeated through the image of terror. In this sense every painter could be considered a Perseus, and Caravaggio painted a Medusa. Did not Freud (1940 [1922]) say that the representation of Medusa's head, with its phallic abundance, helped to deny castration anxiety in the confrontation with the female sex and consequently with the difference between the sexes? We see that, at least for Caravaggio, the first image that confronts the subject with the difference between the sexes produces terror or, in psychoanalytic terms, produces a disruptive effect (Benyakar, 2005) in human beings, provoking a potentially traumatic affect that forces the psyche to work on the lifelong Oedipus complex.

The representation is given to us by pure immediate perception—more precisely, it is a conquest for Enaudeau, who cites Green (1987), when he writes: "Psychoanalysis is a work on representations (unconscious and preconscious) that, at least in certain cases, becomes a labour of representation" (Enaudeau, 1998, p. 141).

I suggest that, even though the genesis of the judgment of existence follows that of attribution, it re-signifies the latter *après-coup*, and the ego's initial good and bad pleasure–again becomes good or bad *après-coup* in function of the judgment of existence as filtered through the Oedipus complex.

My hypothesis is that the possibility of creativity in both sexes involves the possibility to sustain within the psyche a never resolved tension between the *phallic order* and the *nothingy order*, forces in tension whose dynamics and fluidity determine whether the subject will exhibit greater or less porosity in the work of representing into which the streams of all psychic agencies flow, both in the work of representation and in the vicissitudes of the concomitant affect. Two images provoke questions in human beings and produce a more or less traumatic effect, depending on the individual. One is an image we have never experienced and from which we have been excluded forever: the primal scene. "We originate in a scene we were never in: an image lacking in human beings," states Pascal Quignard (1994, p. 22). The other is the image of the difference between the sexes confronting which is inevitable. Both provoke questions in human beings throughout their lives. I cite a passage from Quignard that I consider most revealing of the work of representing human beings:

> Whether they close their eyes or dream at night, open their eyes or closely observe real things in light shed by the sun, whether their gaze wanders afar or is lost, whether they turn their eyes to the book in their hands, whether sitting in the dark they watch the development of a film or let themselves be absorbed in the contemplation of a painting, human beings have a desiring gaze that is seeking another image behind everything they see. (Quignard, 1994, p. 34).

I would add that, in my opinion, this work of representation, which is the core of all psychic work of working through, is also the core of every creative process. When I refer to "work," I am not referring only to the sustained labor involved in creative activity, in the solitude of the studio or when facing the anxiety of the blank page, but in particular the psychic work that supports it as a base. This base is not static or immobile, nor a fixed baseboard of creativity, forever given. Like a moving sculpture, or even more, like interactive art, in which the spectator is both passive and active in relation to the work of art, in the creative subject the life drive (desire to desire) and death drive (desire to not desire), the psychic agencies, the multiple sexual identifications, passivity and activity, libido and inertia, all interact and converse with each other. Here, Eros finally triumphs, having succeeded in deactivating traumatic effraction and transforming it into the sensuality of a text, the palette of colors in a painting, or the movement that animates a sculpture.

Murielle Gagnebin (1994) suggests approaching the work of art avoiding any pathography or psychobiography of the author; she proposes, instead, four metapsychological causes that enable the work of art to emerge: (1) the artist's capital of drive: "the richer and more available it is, the denser the work will be materially" (p. 31); (2) the working through of absence; (3) the artist's possibility to introject harmonious bisexuality; and (4) the sublimation of part drives. The free circulation of these four causes determines the poietic of the work of art, but, she states, not so much in an act of sublimation, as in a movement of metonymic displacement or perhaps of reaction formation.

Didier Anzieu (1981) considers that in the author pierced through by creation, psychic work is similar to dream work or the work of mourning. What is common to these three is that they constitute phases of crisis for the psychic apparatus. He draws a distinction between creativity, which is within the reach of many, and creation, characterized by contributing something new (something never done before) and by public recognition, sooner or later, of the creator's work. Anzieu attributes the larger numbers of male creators compared to female creators to the struggle against death that is creation, in which men, unable to engender, find compensation for their desire to transcend. However, he suggests a hypothesis that interests me: that creation involves a combination of the maternal, the paternal, the feminine, may and the masculine, but also the sexually indeterminate. The creator is one "who has free play of all the variables of the sexual in thought and who has the luck or intelligence to use at the right moment whatever is required in each phase of the work" (Anzieu, 1981, p. 19).

Traditionally, women are assigned the place of the muse of the creating man, and in figurative art in particular, the place of the model: the beautiful, the voluptuous, or the uncanny. As highlighted by Marian Cao (2000), the history of art, through the representation of the woman, has expressed a certain conception of the woman and has denied women: "The different vanguards have treated the image of the woman either as part of a landscape, irreducible to itself—as in Fauvism, Cubism and Surrealism—or as the vampires, a threatening spider that weaves its web to eat the man" (Cao, 2000, p. 23). In the images of abductions and rapes, Cao continues, "that plague Western imaginary, women do not appear as victims, but as voluptuous, lascivious beings" (p. 25). These images have passed on into publicity, which drinks from sources of artistic iconography that remain alive. In iconographic representation, the woman is either viewed directly or is looking at herself in a mirror.

Many creative women were recognized because they were someone's daughter, as was the painter Artemisia Gentileschi, at the beginning, or somebody's lover, as in the case of the sculptor Camille Claudel. It took Frida Kahlo great courage to make her work be valued independently of her husband, Diego Rivera. However, as Cao stresses, when we read about Frida Kahlo, the sad and tragic facts tend to overshadow the definition of her works. Maria Sklodowska, in spite of having won two Nobel Prizes, one in physics and the other in chemistry, was better known by the name of her husband, Mr. Curie.

Many paintings by Artemisia Gentileschi were attributed to her father or to Caravaggio, not to mention the public humiliation and tortures to which she was subjected after being raped. In the anthological exhibition of her work, held in Florence in 1991 (cited by Cao, 2000, p. 35), the catalogue stated: "Proven and truly exceptional mastery for a womanish brush," only to add "Artemisia, lascivious and precocious young woman"—an incredible summation of prejudices and injuries on the creative condition of women. I quote Lacan when he says, in a subtle and evocative play on words: "on la *dit-femme*, on la *diffâme*" (you call her woman and you defame her) (Lacan, 1972–73, p. 79).

The psychic topics need to enter into an effervescent tension if creativity is to emerge. However, the necessary condition for this is the production of a fertile subjectivation—it is in the conquest of her condition as subject, in her ability to run through drive circuits fluidly, to oscillate past the "three modalities of satisfaction, the active, the auto-erotic and passivation" (Penot, 2006, p. 1590) described by Penot. This subjectivation cannot be attained if social and cultural conditions are unfavorable: the ego and its circumstances, in the words of the philosopher José Ortega y Gasset. I am sure that for creativity to emerge freely from the unconscious, certain trans-subjective social circumstances are also required.

Concerning the subjectivation that is necessary as a conquest, some words follow about a contemporary artist who is of great interest for psychoanalysis, since she accompanies her work with letters, notebooks, and commentary, sometimes on the back of her drawings, describing her states of humor and feelings during her creative process—works primarily conceived by work of subjectivation, achieved by means of her art and her personal analysis in a highly intricate way. I am referring here to the painter and sculptor Louise Bourgeois.

Thus, we read, in reference to traumatic effraction and her effort at subjectivation:

> I have dragged Louise Bourgeois around with me for over forty years. Each day I brought her wound along with me and I have carried my wounds ceaselessly, without rest, like a piece of leather with holes in it that cannot be repaired. I am a collection of wooden pearls forever unstrung. [Bourgeois, 2011, p. 4]

In one of her notes, she summarizes the place of the death drive in all works: in sculpture, voluntarist attempts lead to formlessness or incoherence.

> Sculpture may incorporate a lot of blind and formless aggression, but it demands more than that—aggression is necessary and useful, but not sufficient. Although rage leads to destruction, sustained fury may be productive. [Bourgeois, 2011, p. 65]

Perhaps she is speaking of the need of the death drive in the creative act that destroys forms and allows Eros to generate other representations more concordant with the working through of the traumatic, that we proposed at the beginning of this chapter. In a humorous vein, Bourgeois describes the involvement of the drive and the body, sometimes laid bare, in view of the artist's perceptual intensity in relation to the world, and the way it is transformed into representation: "luckily, we have only five senses, what a lot of problems and suffering this saves us! Imagine if we had fourteen!" (Bourgeois, 2011, p. 72).

"Being-in-the-world means," in the thinking of Emanuelle Coccia (2010), "above all, *being* in the sensitive, moving in it, doing or undoing it without interruption" (p. 10), I believe that there is no creativity without suffering during the creative process, whether in the writer's confrontation with the blank page, the painter's with the empty canvas, and the sculptor's with formless matter. The elusive is the adequate expression of suffering, since it puts artists in contact with their own penury in relation to the magnitude of the senses. Perhaps also because the contact with the primary process demanded by creativity is a source of anxiety, censure is not lifted without consequences.

I do not draw conclusions; I do, however, insist that for creativity to emerge, in men or in women, their psychic agencies and repression need to be porous enough and the dialogue between their life and death drives needs to be free of fear, for their multiple identifications, feminine or masculine or indeterminate, to refract freely, for the psychic work of working through the traumatic to find a livable and fertile solution in creative work.

I will let Louise Bourgeois be my spokesperson in closing:

> The work of art is barely acting-out, not understanding. If we understood it, there would no longer be any need to create the work. [Bourgeois, 2011, p. 81]

References

Alizade, M. (1992). Nada de mujer. In: *La sensualidad femenina* (pp. 27–65). Buenos Aires: Amorrortu.

Anzieu, D. (1981*). Le corps de l'oeuvre*. Paris: Gallimard.

Benjamin, J. (1995). *Like Subjects, Love Objects: Essays on Recognition and Sexual Difference*. New Haven, CT: Yale University Press. (Spanish translation by Jorge Pitiagorsky. Buenos Aires: Paidos, 1997.)

Benyakar, M. (2005). *Lo traumático*. Buenos Aires: Editorial Biblos.

Bourgeois, L. (2011). *El retorno de lo reprimido*. Catalogue of the Exhibition of Works of Art and Writing of Louise Bourgeois organized by Fundación Proa, Buenos Aires.

Cao, M. L. F. (2000). La creación artística. Un difícil sustantivo femenino. In: *Creación artística y mujeres* (pp. 23–36). Madrid: Narcea Editorial.

Chaboudez, G. (1994). *Le concept du phallus dans ses articulations lacaniennes*. Paris: Lysimaque.

Coccia, E. (2010). *La vida sensibile*. Spanish trans. by M. T. Mezza. Buenos Aires: Marea Editorial.

Durrmeyer, L. (1999). Et changer de plaisir. In: *La féminité autrement* (pp. 15–25). Paris: PUF.

Enaudeau, C. (1998). *Là-bas comme ici. Le paradoxe de la représentation*. Paris: Gallimard.

Freud, S (1924). The dissolution of the Oedipus complex. In: *Standard Edition, Vol. 19*. London: Hogarth Press.

Freud, S. (1925a). Negation. In: *Standard Edition, Vol. 19*. London: Hogarth Press.

Freud, S. (1925b). Some psychical consequences of the anatomical distinction between the sexes. In: *Standard Edition, Vol. 19*. London: Hogarth Press.

Freud, S. (1940 [1922]). Medusa's head. In: *Standard Edition, Vol. 18*. London: Hogarth Press.

Gagnebin, M. (1994). *Pour une esthétique psychanalytique*. Paris: PUF.

Glocer-Fiorini, L. (2001). *Lo femenino y el pensamiento complejo*. Buenos Aires: Lugar Editorial. (English translation, *Deconstructing the Feminine*. London: Karnac, 2010.)

Green, A. (1987). La représentation de chose entre pulsion et langage. In: *Propédeutique (la métapsychologie revisitée)* (pp. 135–155). Paris: Champ Vallon, 1995.

Heidegger, M. (2000). *Qué es la metafísica?* Spanish translation by H. Cortez & A. Leyte. Madrid: Editorial Alianza.

Horney, K. (1967). *La psychologie de la femme*. French translation. Paris: Payot, 1969.

Lacan, J. (1972–1973). *Le séminaire, Livre XX, Encore*. Paris: Seuil, 1975.

Morin, E. (2007). *Introduction to Complex Thinking*. Porto Alegre: Sulina.

Penot, B. (2006). La position féminine dans les échanges premiers. *Revue Française de Psychanalyse, 70*: 1585–1593.

Pergaud, L. (1912). *La Guerre des Boutons*. Paris: Gallimard, 1994.

Quignard, P. (1994*). Le sexe et l'effroi*. Paris: Gallimard.

Shakespeare, W. (1600). *Much Ado About Nothing*. In: *The Complete Plays of William Shakespeare* (pp. 110–132). New York: Chatham River Press, 1984.

Tesone, J.-E. (2006). La divine jouissance. Le narcissisme féminin et les mystiques. *Revue Française de Psychanalyse, 70*: 1523–1528.

Part III

Yes, we see, but what?
What we hear

14 Hysteria's contribution to subjectivity*

In the hospice of the Salpêtrière lived around five thousand women, most of them indigent, with the most varied pathologies. When Charcot took over in 1871—the first chair in the world of neurology, in the so-called epileptic pavilion of the hospital—the patients were mostly women, with the most varied neurological diagnoses. Charcot knew how to differentiate hysteria in this amalgam of pathological pictures, and by naming it, he gave it an existence of its own (Didi-Huberrman, 1982). To visually document hysteria, he created an *ad-hoc* photography laboratory led by A. Londe, who was to be part of the history of photography. He conceived a photo-electric machine specially designed to capture movement. One of his assistants, Marey, created a procedure called chronophotography, which allowed movement to be broken down and captured in several successive shots during an attack.

Upon entering the hospital, the patient was photographed, and again at the time of a hysterical attack. With this panoply of images, how can we not be tempted to create some hysterical crisis? Between the interest of doctors thirsty for hysterical attacks and patients endowed with an inexhaustible bodily expressiveness, a spiral of surprising mutual enjoyment was formed, to such an extent that some hospitalized patients could have 60 attacks per day.

One of Charcot's assistants, Paul Richer, professor of anatomy at the School of Fine Arts, drew the various stages of the great attack, thus specifying its aesthetics. As a sculptor, he captured patients of the service in stone (Trillat, 1986). In the amphitheater where he made the presentation of the hysterics, Charcot wore clogs, apron, and hat, vestiges of the initial use of this amphitheater as an anatomy room. The famous Tuesday lessons, which Freud would later translate into German, summoned numerous disciples from all over the world. During this presentation of patients—a

* "Hysteria: In memoriam?" APSA Congress 2014, international panel organized by the "Psychoanalysis in Psychiatry" Section of the World Psychiatric Association (WPA). Posted in *SYNOPSIS*, Vol. 27, No. 54, p. 19.

DOI: 10.4324/9781032647791-18

presentation that Lacan was to reproduce in the best French style at the St. Anne Hospital—Charcot, to the rhythm of the tam tam and some luminous rays, hypnotized the patients.

It thus created a great optical machinery through which observation, description in images, or simply of the imaginary, would create certainty. Apparently, it was enough to observe, describe, and photograph, in order to understand. However—something to which Freud was to be sensitive during his stay—for the first time in the history of medicine, and, Charcot creates or suppresses bodily symptoms of conversion through hypnosis exclusively through the word. The word becomes flesh in the body of the hysterical, which used her body to relieve the psyche.

Jean Martin Charcot invited to his private residence every Tuesday night—an extension of his classic Tuesday Lessons—the academic world of the time. The staging of the amphitheater at the hospital had some similarity to the staging at his private *hôtel*—as the large residences were called—located at number 217 Boulevard Saint Germain. It currently houses the Latin American Cultural Center, the most important Latin American cultural center in Paris. Premonitory sign or simple coincidence, during his stay in La Salpêtrière, from September 1885 to February 1886, Freud stayed in a small hotel in Le Goff Street, in the 5th arrondissement in Paris, currently called Hôtel du Brésil.

Charcot rediscovered hysteria, and his work is foundational. About what? By naming hysteria, he separated it from epilepsy and so many other mental alienations, that he managed to isolate it as a nosological entity. Although the term became well known, his studies of the body of hysterics are mostly visual. The symptoms are, above all, visible signs in a body that asked only to be looked at, already a glimpse of the phallic value in hysteria. Charcot described the hysterical attack and divided it into four periods: (1) the first period or epileptoid period, with its three phases: tonic, clonic, and muscle resolution; (2) the second period or clowning, with its phases of contortions and large movements; (3) the third period, of passionate attitudes; and finally (4) the fourth period of hallucinations.

He thus described an order, and although he recognized that hysterical disorders were of psychic origin, unlike Babinsky, he had an organo-dynamic conception of hysteria: he made the psychic disorder depend on a functional location in the brain. Thus, there is a regulated visibility of the hysterical attack, where a disorder catalogued as demoniac was produced. Charcot introduced an order, but despite having intuited the psychic origin of the symptoms, his therapeutic arsenal remained classically rudimentary, limited to electrotherapy, hydrotherapy, and magnetotherapy—not forgetting the compressor of ovaries in search of the pretended anesthesia to the pain of hysterics, in the so called "scientific" form of medical sadism.

By fixing the hysterical in an image, in a patient without history or desire, he turned her into a petrified statue. Perhaps it was no coincidence that he published, jointly with Paul Richer, *The Demoniacs in Art* (Charcot & Richer, 1887), and that he had as his subtitle, *The Deformed and the Diseases in Art*. Hysteria as a deformity of the spirit, to be excluded from the human world: the Inquisition had long tried to combat hysteria at the stake, with cremation as purification of inadmissible sexuality. But where there was fire, ashes remain: it is well known how important the experience with Charcot and the contact with the body of hysteria was to be for Freud. I won't talk about the double consciousness initially developed with Breuer, and then his discovery of the unconscious.

If I dwell on the pre-psychoanalytic period of hysteria, it is to emphasize that, paradoxically, a certain drift of contemporary psychiatry returns to that stage. The modern sometimes hides a certain archaism. The disappearance of hysteria in the nosography of the *Diagnostic and Statistical Manual of Mental Disorders* (DSM-IV; APA, 1995), which prevails as a reference of psychiatry in the Occident, is not only an innocent sign of the times; it is a reflex that, for the diagnosis of a psychic pathology, a pile of symptoms is taken into account, without correlation with the structure, or worse, without taking into account the dynamics of the underlying psychic functioning.

It can be seen the distance of certain psychiatry in the consideration of the subject. The DSM is defined as a glossary of descriptions based on empirical data. Each mental disorder is there conceptualized as "a clinically significant behavioral or psychological syndrome or pattern that occurs in an individual and that is associated with present distress or disability or with a significantly increased risk of suffering death, pain, disability, or an important loss of freedom" (p. 21).

This use of the DSM as a unit of criteria aims to simplify the complex and thus overwhelms subjectivity. The symptoms are grouped into syndromes, but by a non-innocent slip they become diseases with an entity, which are treated univocally according to the symptomatology and not according to the subjective problem of the patient. As in Charcot's time, the symptom exists and is considered of to be psychic origin, but it is treated according to symptomatic grouping, mainly with psychotropic drugs. The symptom is decapitated, but simultaneously the head is cut off from the metaphor and with it the possibility of symbolic expression of the conflictive.

But I trust in hysteria—in its power to challenge established knowledge, as it has been doing since ancient times. Hysteria has always challenged medicine and the social order, since it touches sexuality and, perhaps, a sexuality even more difficult to admit: a female sexuality (in both sexes) and a desire for enjoyment feared by its unlimited character. The first notions of hysteria date from Egyptian antiquity, the Kahun

Papyrus (1900 BC) already describes the nefarious wanderings of the uterus. Plato, Hippocrates, Galen, and so many others spoke with contempt of hysteria, and religion may pay for its demonic daring at the stake in the Inquisition.

What is it that hysteria defends, if not what led Freud to the discovery of the unconscious and the split subject? That is, considering the subject in its singularity means being able to move from the Charcotian staging to an act of word that returns to its condition of desiring a subject with a particular story that makes it unique. If the subject is treated without them assuming their subjective responsibility for what happens to them, we are depriving them of their condition of being unique and different—that is, of their subjective historicization. The apparent therapeutic success of a certain contemporary psychiatry would then consist in imposing a pharmacological order where symptoms are only conceived as expressions of sterile chaos, without any metaphorical relief.

However, it is in the metaphor of their body that hysteria has always triumphed. Conversion is the symbolic way to express a suffering that has persisted throughout history; it is not easy to neutralize the subjectivity of the hysterical subject, and I bet that the DSM will not silence hysteria—but that is another story. We are currently witnessing a certain claudication of the subjectivity of the psychiatrist and of the transferential relationship, and a neutralization of the patient as subject. The patient is no longer photographed by Charcot's optical machine, although brain images may give the illusion that one day we will see the unconscious, but it is standardized through forms that the patient fills in in the waiting room, thus grouping the symptoms in a diagnosis that only piles them up, leaving their uniqueness excluded.

Charcot showed the hysterical body to exhaustion, but was stuck in his purely visual apprehension of it. Freud, instead, listened to the hysterical subject and allowed them to put into words their singular speech, which led to the discovery of the unconscious. In that sense we owe a lot to Freud, it seems redundant to insist, but we also owe a great deal to hysteria, precious bulwark of the struggle to defend undomesticated subjectivity. Paradoxically, some currents of contemporary psychiatry take the hysterical back to the Charcotian period, by which they recognize symptoms that they pretend to be objectifiable, in the best positivist style, but deny the symptoms their metaphorical value, seeking only a pharmacological erasure of them.

The phrase that maintained that a therapeutic success with an obsessive neurotic was their hysterization—that is, the exit from their representative poverty towards a better symbolic expression of their conflict—hardly circulates among colleagues. I do not idealize hysteria, but I trust that it will once again challenge the established knowledge that historically seeks to deny the split and desiring subject, to rediscover its place. The hysterical is no longer burned, ignored, in a refined form of the cold bonfire of the DSM. In Dante's inferno fire prevailed, but cold zones of freezing also co-existed. The result was similar.

Freud recalls, in his text "On Psychotherapy" (1905):

> Painting, says Leonardo, works *per via di porre*, for it applies a substance—particles of color—where there was nothing before, on the colorless canvas; sculpture, however, proceeds *per via di levare*, since it takes away from the block of stone all that hides the surface of the statue contained in it. In a similar way, the technique of suggestion aims at proceeding *per via di porre*; it is not concerned with the origin, strength and meaning of the morbid symptoms, but instead, it super-imposes something—a suggestion—in the expectation that il will be strong enough to restrain the pathogenic idea coming to expression. Analytic therapy, on the other hand, does not seek to add or to intro-duce anything new, but to take away something, to bring out some-thing; and to this end concerns itself with the genesis of the morbid symptoms and the psychical context of the pathogenic idea which it seeks to remove. [p. **260**]

I believe that hysteria deserves a just tribute as a paradigm of its struggle in defense of subjectivity, and in that sense, it is representative of all psy-chic pathology. As such, it deserves a place that is not only historical, but current, whose understanding is reached, as Freud said, by *via di levare* (revealing metaphorical meanings) and not by *via di porre*. In a reductive way it is this last way that the DSM seem to retake, analogically, to the pre-psychoanalytic stage, in a de-subjectivant crusade, fascinated as they are by the suggestion of symptomatic expression and not by the meta-phorical value of it.

References

APA (1995). *The Diagnostic and Statistical Manual of Mental Disorders (DSM-IV)*. Washington, DC: American Psychiatric Association. (Spanish translation, Bar-celona: Masson.)

Charcot, J.-M., & Richer, P. (1887). *Les démoniaques dans l'art*. Paris: Delayahe et Lecrosmer.

Didi-Huberman, G. (1982). *Invention de l'hystérie*. Paris: Macula.

Freud, S. (1905). On psychotherapy. In: *Standard Edition, Vol. 7* (p. 260). London: Hogarth Press, 1978.

Trillat, E. (1986). *Histoire de l'hystérie*. Paris: Seghers.

Iconography of the Salpêtrière Hospital

In J. M. Charcot's time (Musée de l'Assistance Publique de Paris).

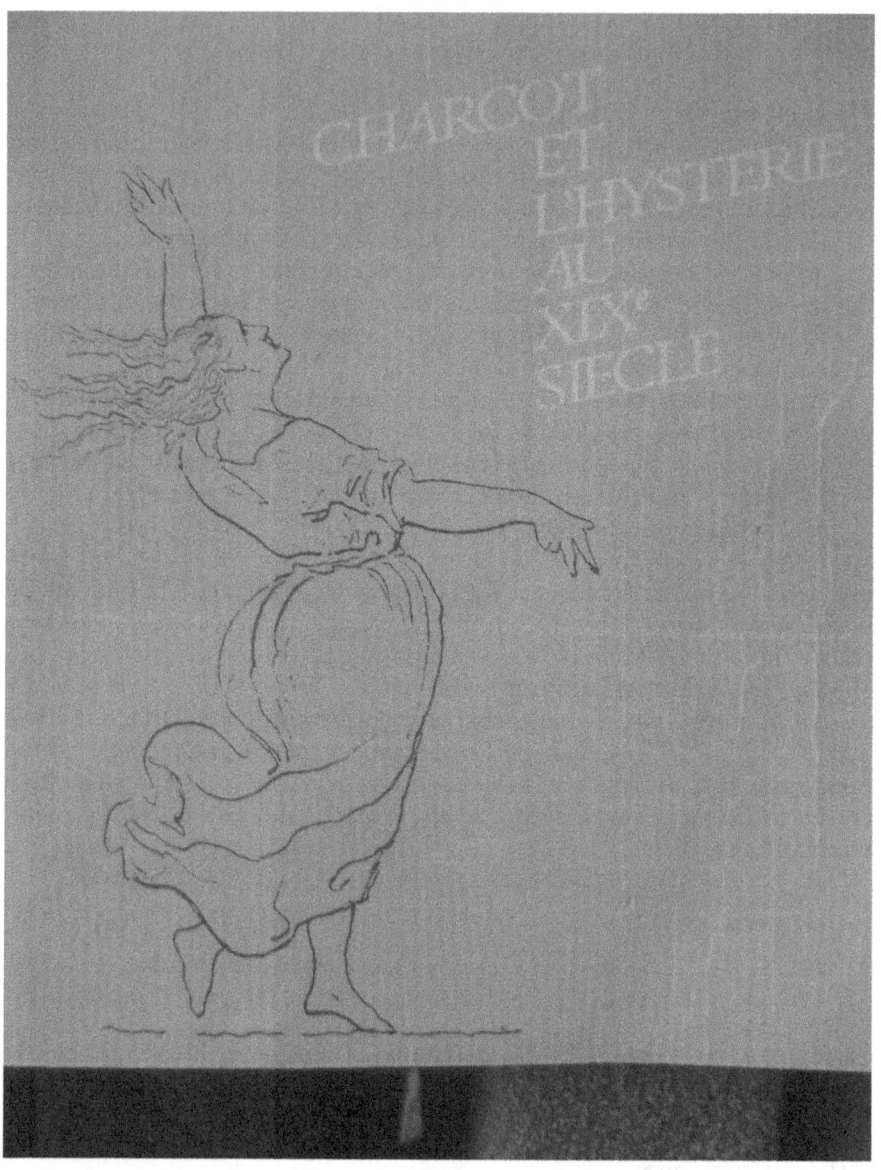

Image 14.1 Charcot and hysteria in the nineteenth century (Museum of Public Assistance of Paris).

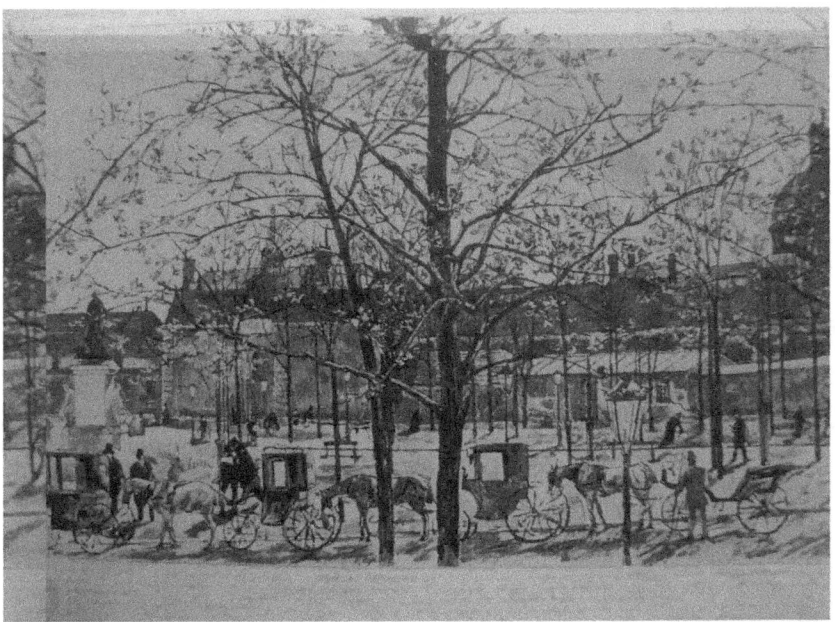

Image 14.2 Iconography of photographs of Professor Charcot's service at La Salpêtrière (Museum of Public Assistance of Paris).

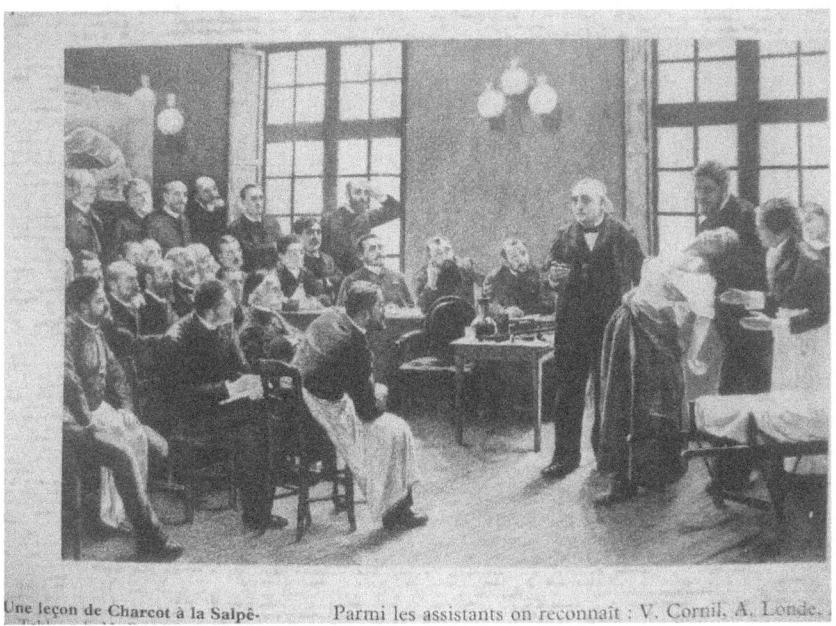

Une leçon de Charcot à la Salpê-   Parmi les assistants on reconnaît : V. Cornil, A. Londe,

Image 14.3 A Charcot lesson at La Salpetriere (Museum of Public Assistance of Paris).

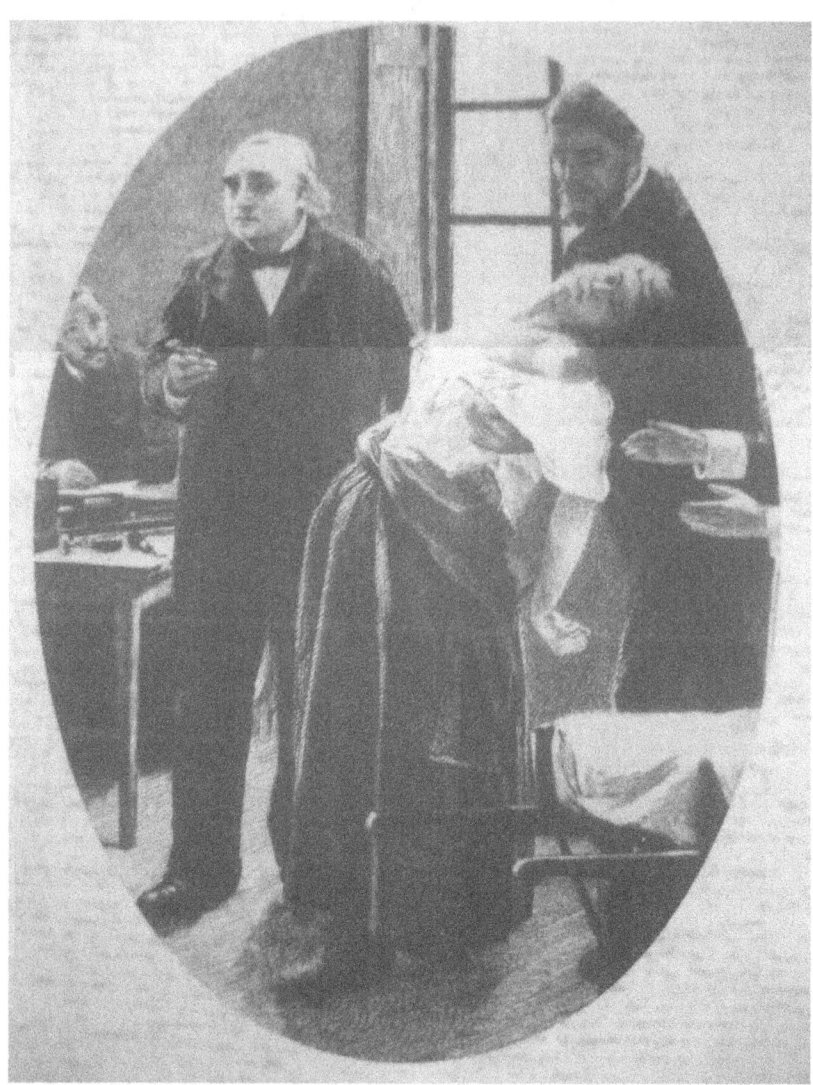

Image 14.4 Iconography of photographs of Professor Charcot's service at La Salpêtrière (Museum of Public Assistance of Paris).

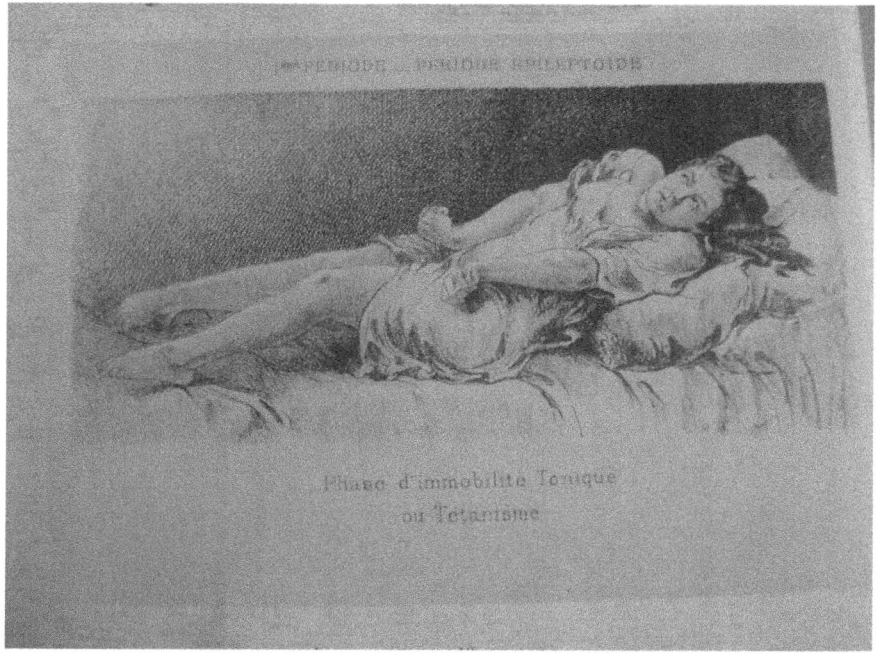

Image 14.5 Phase of tonic immobility or tetanus (Museum of Public Assistance of Paris).

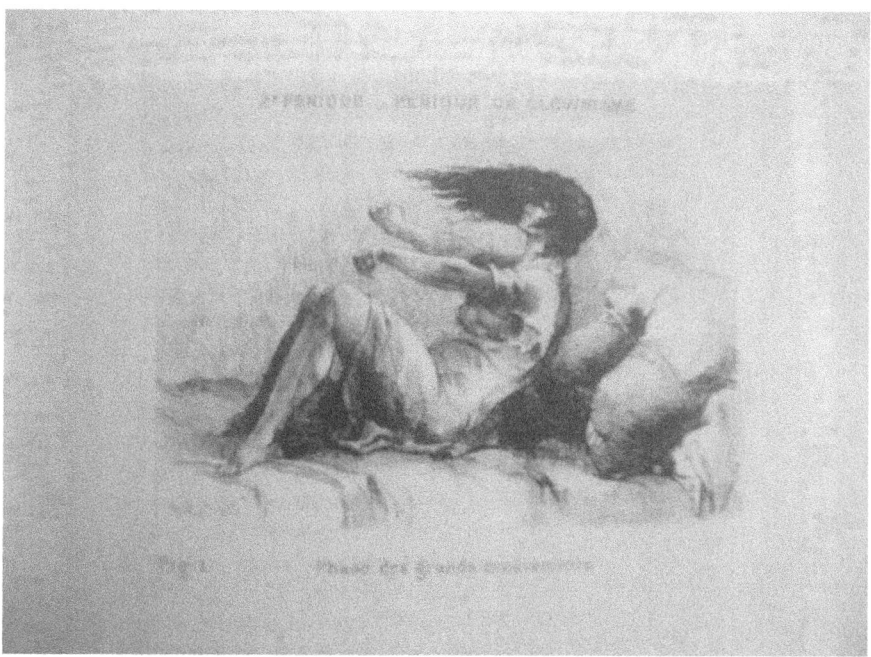

Image 14.6 Large movement phase (Museum of Public Assistance of Paris)

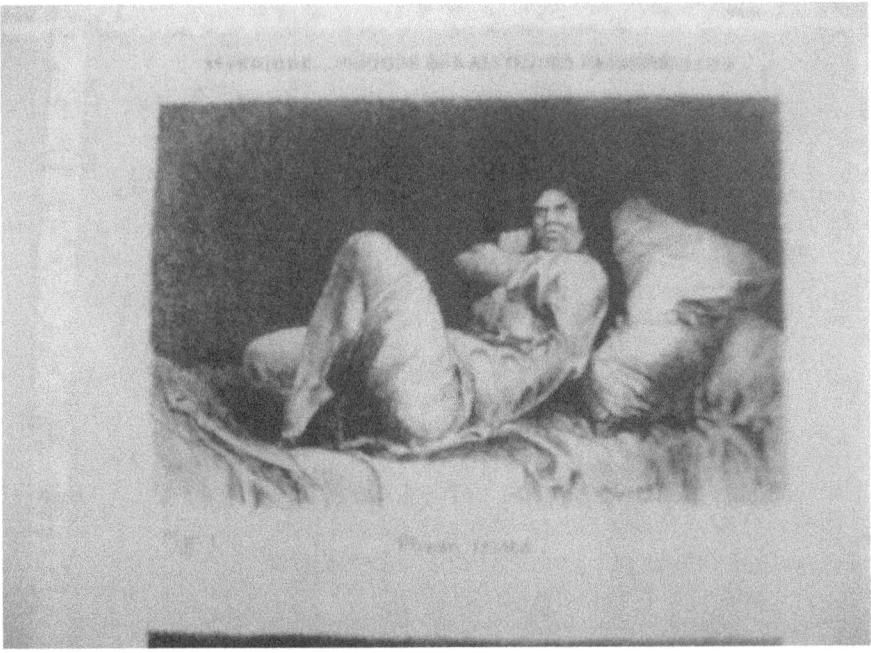

Image 14.7 Sad phase (Museum of Public Assistance of Paris).

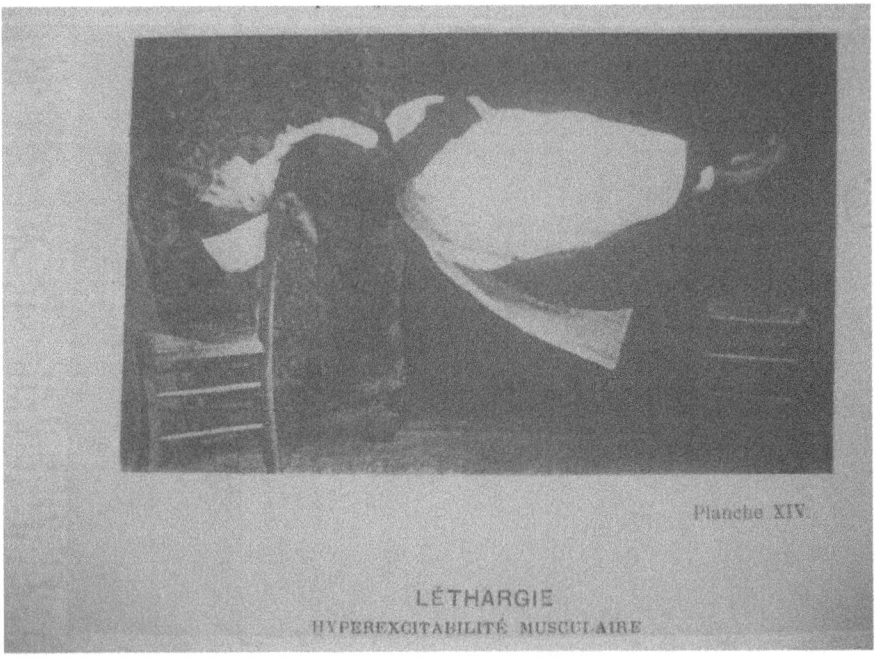

Image 14.8 Lethargy (Museum of Public Assistance of Paris).

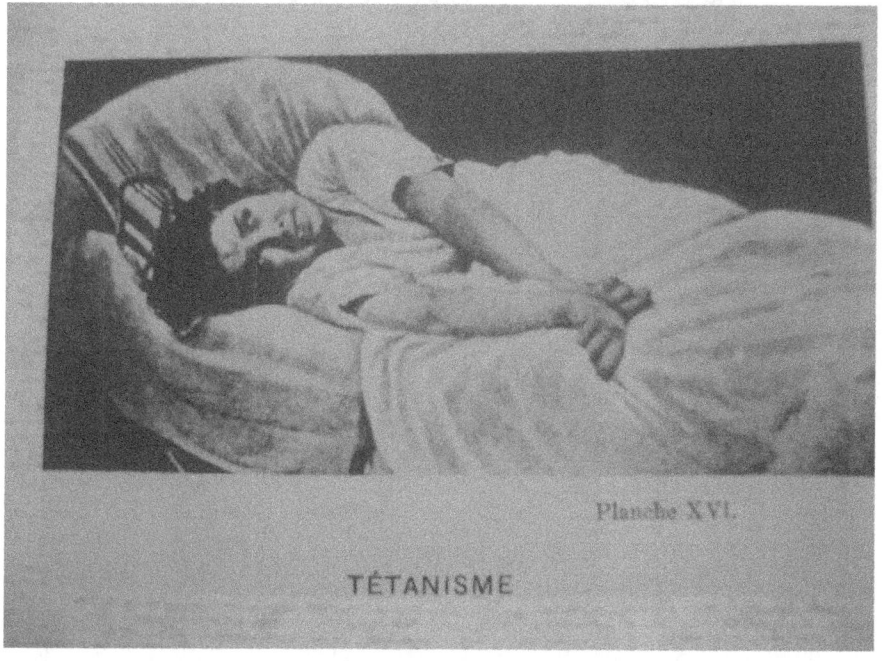

Image 14.9 Tetanus (tonic immobility) (Museum of Public Assistance of Paris).

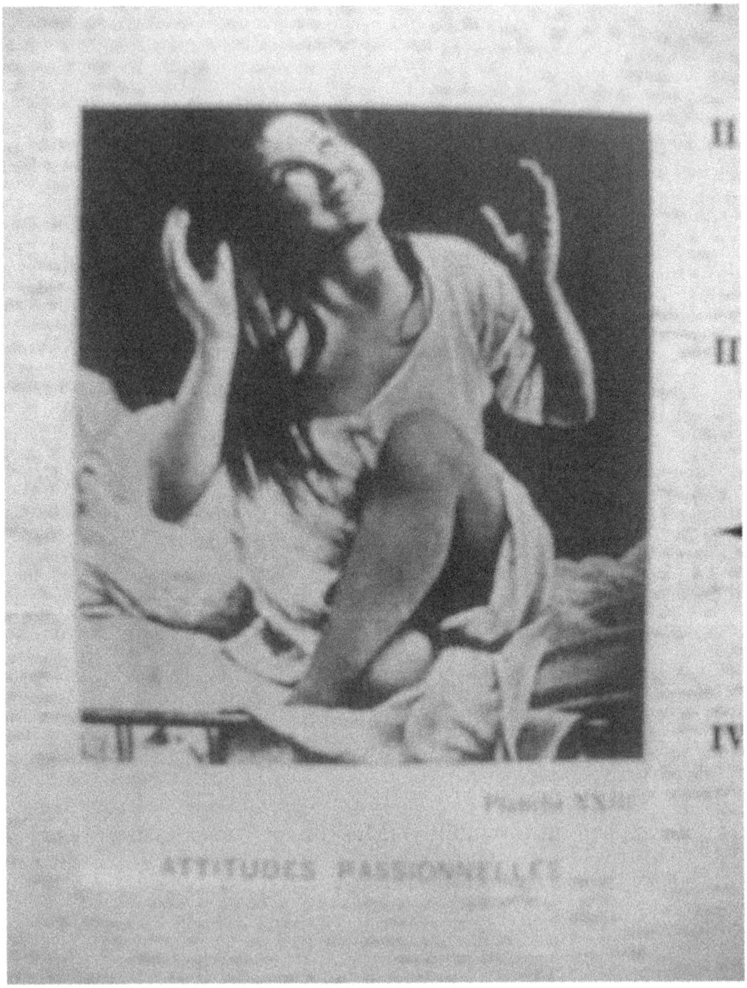

Image 14.10 Passionate attitudes (Museum of Public Assistance of Paris).

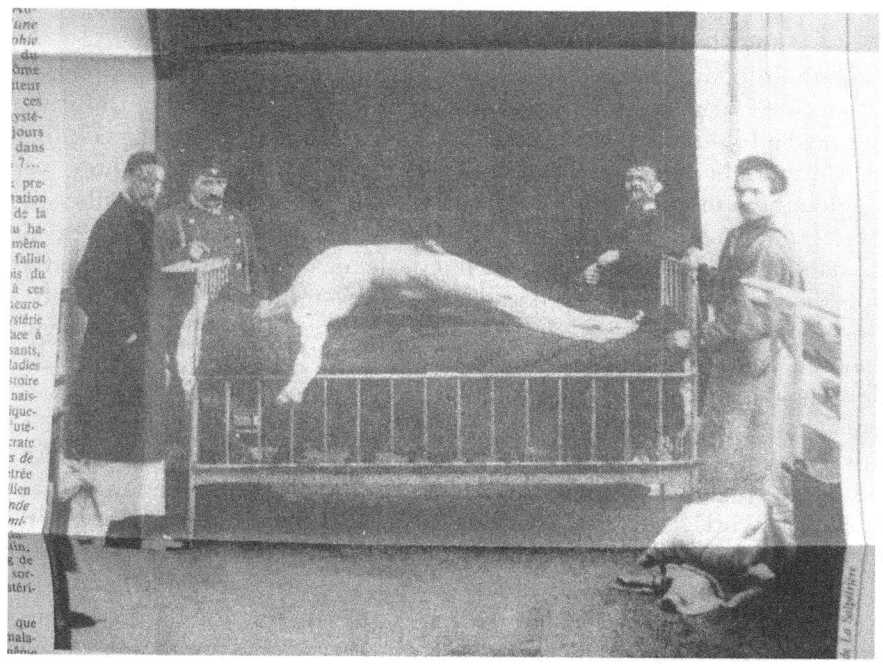

Image 14.11 Iconography of photographs of Professor Charcot's service at La Salpêtrière (Museum of Public Assistance of Paris).

15 Sexes and genders*

The human being is confronted from the beginning with two potential traumatic experiences: On the one hand, the existence of the other, always irreducible to our fantasies, is the first potentially traumatic aspect; the other human beings, our loved ones, are always different from how we imagine them or as we wish they were—without forgetting that other in oneself that constitutes the unconscious. "I am another," said the poet A. Rimbaud (1871). And, on the other hand, the other potentially traumatic aspect is the sexuality of each one, always mysterious in its singularity, which is expressed in psychoanalytic theory as emerging from the drive. It should be noted that the drive is not instinct. The instinct is the same for each species, and is typical of animals. It has cycles in which it is expressed and given by nature. The concept of drive in the human being is different. Freud defines it as a boundary concept between soma and psyche; it is a constant force that knows no cycles. The soma demands that the psyche work constantly. No one escapes dealing with the drive. Even during sleep, the drive does not rest and is expressed in our dreams. The drive can have a range of destinations, ranging from direct satisfaction to sublimation—that is, transformed into a symbolic production that allows a transformation of the direct drive into a creative production of the spirit—like reading, writing, painting, a sport, or any activity that does not require direct satisfaction. But no one escapes the internal stimulus of their drives. In the best of cases one may sublimate them, although it is never possible to sublimate the drives completely: there is always a part of direct satisfaction. The notion of sexuality in Freudian theory is broad, encompassing much more than the genital. But it is always a psychosexuality, and this is fundamental to a differentiation between human sexuality and the sexuality from other living beings. Within sexuality, there is a distinction between oral satisfaction (as in intake of food

* Presented at a Conference at the Argentine Psychoanalytic Association, Extension Course organized by Dr. Mónica Hamra: "Why Do Words Heal?", panel of 18 November 2021.

DOI: 10.4324/9781032647791-19

or of other substances), anal sexuality (as in the expulsion or retention of feces), and genital sexuality itself, whose relative synthesis is reached from puberty on with the possibility of orgasm—without forgetting that the whole body of the human being has an erogenous capacity, even our internal organs.

The great Freudian revolution has been to describe childhood psychosexuality—that is, that existing in the child. He described the sexuality of the child by calling it "perverse-polymorphous," not a very happy expression, but I mention it in case you have heard it. What does Freud mean by this term? That sexuality in humans, unlike in animals, is not determined by nature, but that adult sexuality is an avatar of the evolution of child psychosexuality. Child sexuality that does not disappear with the passage of time; it remains in force in adults—an enigmatic destiny that cannot be predicted, but that concerns the uniqueness of each subject. In that sense, there would be as many possible sexualities as there are subjects. This notion of childhood sexuality was first described by a pediatrician named Samuel Lindner, who observed the pleasure the baby had in sucking (Freud, 1905, p. 179). Freud takes up this idea and develops it. His proposal generated a lot of resistance. For example, his book published in 1905, entitled *Three Essays on the Theory of Sexuality*, where he describes child sexuality (p. 125), had a print run of 1,000 copies and took four years to sell. Sexuality still produces scandals today. We are not in the Victorian era of repression, but the exhibition of sexuality, in its diversity, is still disturbing—not only religions and their prejudices, but even psychoanalytic theory and its own prejudices. No one is left out of sexuality; as a question, it is a permanent question for all human beings.

We have gone from hetero-normative sexuality, to all LGBTI+ movements—lesbian, gay, trans, binary and intersex: diversity that is not exhausted in this listing, as new formulations are constantly emerging. The so-called "new sexualities"—in reality they have always existed, if in a hidden way—have managed to gain a space in society. From shame to pride, movement is pendulous. From the field of mental health, the legitimization of sexual diversities has modified the labels with which traditional psychiatry had tried to classify human beings. Borders are less hermetic, and the notion of perversion has changed (Tesone, 2020). Until not many years ago, perversion was classified according to certain sexual behaviors. Joyce McDougall (1978), a French psychoanalyst of New Zealand origin, proposed several years ago that the notion of perversion should be reserved for pedophiles and rapists. The remaining human sexual behaviors, insofar as they are carried out between consenting adults, are part of the expression of human sexuality, without pathological connotations. In fact, in the DSM, the *Classification Manuals of the American Psychiatric Association*, this term does not appear. Perhaps the case is not the same in the Orient, where some sexual behaviors, are punished with death.

In Christianity, in the nineteenth century, in the convents of France, a book circulated, with an endless list of sins related to sexual behavior, which, although not punishable by death, were obviously forbidden. That book was, incidentally, very coveted by subjects with a lack of imagination. Until now we have been talking about sexuality: sex, but not gender. The word "gender" was introduced, in the Anglo-Saxon world, by John Money in the United States and then by Robert Stoller and appears in the 1950–60s the sex/gender couple. It was stated that sex was biological, whereas gender was socio-cultural. Then it was taken up mainly by feminist movements and sexual minorities.

From psychoanalysis, Laplanche (2003) in his text on "Gender in sexual theory" draws a very interesting distinction between gender, which, being plural, is usually double, masculine–feminine, but it is not so by nature, and sex, which is, on the other hand, dual, both because of sexual reproduction and because of its human symbolization, which fixes that duality in a stereotyped way—that is, presence/absence; phallic/neutered. The sexual-drive is multiple, polymorphous, it is the unconscious residue of the repression-symbolization of gender by sex. The sexual-impulsive, infantile par excellence is a non-procreative sexuality, it is the perverse child: what Laplanche calls enlarged sexuality.

Linked more to the fantasy than to the object itself—that is, to what the subject fantasizes—and not so much to an external object, whether to a shoe in the case of the fetishist or to a person or parts of a person, the sexual-impulsive can therefore be autoerotic, ruled by unconscious fantasy. It precedes the differentiation of sexes, even genders; it is oral, anal, and genital. Laplanche reframes the enigma of femininity–masculinity: it is not purely biological, nor purely psychological or socio-cultural, but a mixture of the three. It is more important to think that what defines gender is the existence of the other and their assignment. The assignment indicates the priority of the other in the process. That other arises from the small group of the close family and affective environment that inscribes that *microsocius*; it is not about society as a whole. In this sense, there would be a precedence of gender with respect to sex, depending on the precedence of the assignment with respect to symbolization: identification first, not to the adult, but by the adult. This highlights the contingent, perceptive, illusory character of the anatomical differentiation of sex. Until this theorizing, sexuality had been conceived as binary, whether sex or gender was taken into account. We are currently witnessing a gender called "fluid," by which the person does not identify with any sex or any gender but oscillates, deconstructing binarity and claiming an oscillating or, rather, neutral identity.

The choice is not to choose; there is a blurring of boundaries between sexes and genders. The person does not feel as belonging to any traditional category and chooses his love object based on the condition of another person who attracts them, not based on their belonging to a type of binarism. Fluidity allows you to oscillate in your object choices. From affirmed sexual identity, we have moved on to an oscillating identity, with porous and easily traversable borders. We move away from the category currently called cisgender—that is, as recognized as the gender that corresponds to a biological sex.

In reality, there are several factors that determine biological sex, and these are not exclusively attributable to the difference between male and female. The Italian political philosopher, Lorenzo Bernini (2017) (whose work we will quote extensively) summarizes them as follows:

1. *Sex chromosomes:* Beyond the standard configurations of masculine (XY) and feminine (XX), there are others, such as XXY, XO, XX–XY (which contemporary medicine classifies, respectively, as Klinefelter syndrome, Turner syndrome, and sexual mosaicism).
2. *Sex hormones:* Female (estrogen) and male (androgen) hormones are actually present in different percentages in all humans, and their production and assimilation during pregnancy, during infancy, and after adolescence can give rise to physical constitutions (called "sexual phenotypes") that are typically feminine, or masculine, or atypical with respect to the standards of feminine and masculine.
3. *The external genitalia:* Also in this case, in addition to the scrotum and penis, vulva and clitoris, there are atypical organs with respect to the standards of the feminine and the masculine: for example, erectile organs of dimensions and intermediate aspect somewhere between the penis and the clitoris (which medicine often insists on wanting to define as "micro-penis" or "hypertrophied clitoris").
4. *The internal genitalia:* In contrast to the position of the standard masculine and feminine organs, not only the vagina, uterus and ovaries, but also the testicles can be contained inside the abdomen; In addition, not all vaginas flow into a uterus, and not all are deep enough to be penetrated by an erect medium-sized penis.

Before approaching this debate, however, we have to equip ourselves not only with an appropriate "vocabulary," but also with an adequate "grammar," questioning the terms and rules of our pre-understanding of sexuality, says Bernini. For example, it is difficult to get out of the binary conception, to the point that bisexuality is usually considered not as a third sexual orientation, but as the sum of the other two—not to mention the genetic category of intersex, either XO or XXY, or other multiple possibilities of the so-called "anomalies"—actually genetic variants, always interesting to take into account as modalities of the human.

Bernini argues that the feeling of belonging to a socially recognizable category of person identifies him or her as a cisgender man or woman, or as transgender (who recognizes himself or herself in the opposite gender to his biological sex, or in an intermediate gender between masculine and feminine), fluid gender (who sometimes feels masculine, sometimes feminine), gender indeterminate (uncertain), a-gender (neither masculine nor feminine), genderqueer or genderfuck (consciously or provocatively hostile to the standards of masculine and feminine).

Likewise, Bernini differentiates the gender role—that is, the external manifestation of gender according to social conventions—as potentially masculine, feminine, or androgynous; of the registered gender, i.e., the gender mark as recorded in the registry office and in official documents. While gender identity, gender role, and registered gender may be consistent with each other, they are not necessarily so. There are therefore several possibilities of gender expression—as many as result from the multiple possible combinations of gender identity, gender role, and registered gender. These may also remain unchanged over time, or they may change throughout the life of a subject. But even knowing all this, contemporary psychology still continues to use gender in the first instance as a binary concept that, reflecting the difference between the sexes, is exhausted in the alternative between the masculine and the feminine.

The sex–gender–sexual orientation classification system is, therefore, Bernini asserts, imperfect, insufficient, and contradictory; it and produces "ideal types" ("the Man," "the Woman," but also "the Heterosexual," "the Homosexual"…), which are sometimes far from the experience lived by the subjects that should be described from this system. The challenge is, as suggested by Diana Maffia (2010), "to face the body of another (another or other) not as a physical body, but as a lived body." And she proposes a symbolic border that does not separate, but that is a meeting place, and not a struggle for hegemonic power. Sexual difference, says Joan W. Scott, "constitutes an insoluble dilemma, and is open to all kinds of variations in the way it is lived" (Scott, 2012; quoted by Laufer, 2022). As Scott recalls, quoting Lacan (1964): "in psychism, there is nothing by which the subject can be placed as a male or as a feminine." Therefore, body, sex, and sexuality remain undisciplined; they do not simply fall into binary categories (Laufer, 2022). And these are some of today's complex questions about human sexuality.

References

Bernini, L. (2017). *Las teorías queer*. Barcelona: Editorial Egales.
Freud, S. (1905). *Three Essays on the Theory of Sexuality. Standard Edition, Vol. 7*, p. 125, London: Hogarth Press, 1978.
Lacan, J. (1964). *Le séminaire, Livre XI. Les quatre concepts fondamentaux de la psychanalyse*. Paris: Seuil, 1973.
Laplanche, J. (2003). Le genre, le sexe, le sexual. In: *Libres cahiers pour la psychanalyse. Études sur la théorie de la seduction*. Paris: In Press.
Laufer, L. (2022). *Vers une psychanalyse émancipée*. La Paris: découverte.

McDougall, J. (1978). *Plaidoyer pour une certaine anormalité*. Paris: Gallimard, 1978.

Maffía, D. (2010). Filosofía, política, identidad de género; In: *Un cuerpo. Mil sexos.* Buenos Aires: Topía.

Money, J. (1969). *Transexualism and sex reassignment*. Baltimore: Johns Hopkins Press.

Rimbaud, A. (1871). Lettres du voyant. In: Œuvres completes. Paris: Gallimard, 2009.

Scott, J. W. (2012). *De l'utilité du genre*. Paris: Fayard.

Stoller, R. (1968). *Sex and gender*. NY: Science House.

Tesone, J.-E. (2020). *Revisitando la sexuación*. Symposium of the Asociación Psicoanalítica Argentina, "Tiempos de incertidumbre," 14 November.

16 Cumulative trauma and *"troumatique"**

Freud never abandoned his theory of neurosis—that is, the idea that a traumatic core can be at the origin of every symptom. In the pre-psychoanalytic stage, it was enough to remember it, to remove that foreign body, so that the symptom disappeared. Then came the defense neuroses, and the metaphor of the foreign body spread: it was enough to decrease the defenses in order to arrive, by associative way, to the traumatic scenes—a fact of the external world made irruption in the psyche, causing consequences in the form of symptoms.

However, reality has its subjective nuances. Already in the "Project for a Scientific Psychology," Freud (1950 [1895]) intuited the first lie of hysterics, the *proton pseudos*, and the notion of *"nachträglich"* was inexorably associated with the notion of trauma. Here the translations got themselves in a twist, since they have induced different theorizations. Strachey translated into English as *"deferred action."* López Ballesteros translated it into Spanish as *"a posteriori,"* and in the Amorrortu edition (Buenos Aires) it was translated as *"with delayed effect."* In all of them, a linear temporal causality is maintained: the temporality of the almanac. For Ferenczi, the trauma is closer to the *"deferred action,"* a scene that comes from the outside, hits only once, and acts as a time bomb, but in linear time: its explosion will occur later, without resignification. It is closer to a pre-psychoanalytic conception of trauma.

In French, on the other hand, it was translated as *"après-coup,"* reworked by Lacan, who gave all its density to a temporality with double- or triple-directional meaning, in a mutual resignification. The notion of *après-coup* condenses into a paradoxical movement that secondary logic does not consider—that is, simultaneity, excluding contradiction. The past does not condition the present nor the present the past, it is in the interrelation between the two that there is an absent sense open to the future.

* Cumulative Trauma and Dissociation of the SELF", international panel of the Psychoanalysis and Psychiatry Section of the World Psychiatric Association, within the framework of the 35th Congress of the APSA (Argentine Congress of Psychiatry), April 27–30, 2022—Mar del Plata, Argentina.

DOI: 10.4324/9781032647791-20

Freud described the case of Emma (of whom he speaks in the "Project", and who consulted him when she was 18 years old, as she could not enter the stores). She remembered that, when she walked into a store at age 12, there were men laughing, and she thought her dress was being made fun of. One of the men was sexually attractive to her. Then she remembered that, at the age of 8, she walked into a bakery, and a man, laughing, pinched her genitals through her dress. Freud calls Scene 1, when the child was 8 years old, and Scene 2, when she was 12. Jacques André, on the other hand, places the first time in Scene 2 and the second time in Scene 1, that is, he inverted the notion of chronological temporality. Between the two scenes, the emergence of puberty and sexuality assigns a different meaning to Scene 1 with the 8-year-old. The notion of *après-coup* is highlighted by the theory of seduction.

The *après-coup* not only reverses the chronology, it messes it up. This resignification was conceived from Letter 52 to Fliess (6 December 1896), when Freud anticipated the functioning of the psychic apparatus:

As you know, I am working on the assumption that our psychical mechanism has come into being by a process of stratification: the material present in the form of memory-traces being subjected from time to time to a *re-arrangement* in accordance with fresh circumstances— to a *re-transcription*. [Freud, 1950 [1892–1899], p. 233]

The *après-coup* vacillates between two tensions: brute, disruptive violence on the one hand, and the subtlety of a rewriting on the other, an asymptotic complexity, never finished. But there is no *après* [after] without *coup* [blow]. Now, for Freud and Green and Lacan, the most violent part of the blow comes from within the subject. The memory does not come the way it was produced by the event, but sifted through the associative system of the person, which re-produces it or, rather, produces it again, in a collision between the outside and the interior. In Emma's case, the association is given by dress and laughter.

Although the traumatic experience can be triggered by an event, and in that sense it is conjunctural to what is lived at a given moment in a person's life, it always finds an echo in what I would dare to call the structural poles of every traumatic experience of a subject. Every subject confronts two traumatic aspects inherent in the human condition: that is, to their own sexuality and to the existence of the other.

If our sexuality were predetermined for the species, as instinct is for animals, we would not confront sexual diversity, the object would not be contingent, and our identities would not be wavering. Eros does not leave us in peace: our restlessness does not come only from the death drive. The multiple psychic conflicts that arise from the encounter between drives and the external world begin from the first sensual encounter between the baby and the breast.

In my opinion, when a person is confronted with a disruptive event of any kind, the structural traumatogenic poles of the subject are reactivated—that is, their sexuality and the relationship with the other. Like Russian dolls, they are in-castrated. The threat of castration is always latent.

The field of the traumatic examines, in a paradigmatic way, the unrepresentable, putting in tension the classic analytic device of making the unconscious conscious, revealing that in the analytic session the lifting of repression is not enough to trace something anemic to become mnemic. The traumatic experience occasionally generates a vacuum of figuration that aims at every possible form of representation. What inscription does the perception of the disruptive fact acquire? My purpose will be to open a path rather than indicate an itinerary regarding this question.

"Her childhood had hurt her to such an extent that she could not evoke it," suggests Pascal Quignard (1998, p. 18) of Némie, the protagonist of his novel, *Vie Secrète*. And, I add, perhaps because pain can destroy the possibility of representing it: non-figuration as a defense against unspeakable pain. "What pain does he talk to me about, if I didn't feel it...?" It could be the eloquent phrase of this extreme resource of psychism.

Marguerite Duras says of Lol V. Stein, in her homonymous novel "suffering had not found in her where to slip" (1964, p. 36). And, later in the same novel, he asks: What does suffer without a subject mean? (p. 54)

It is well known that traumatic are disruptive experiences, as suggested by Moty Benyakar: having failed, the ligation processes could not be represented (Benyakar & Lezica, 2005). Outside the figurative, the representable, the traumatic experience escapes the domain of the symbolic and therefore remains suspended in a fixed, stopped, unworkable time. The disruptive effects that are repeated over time in the form of cumulative trauma, trivialized as a daily occurrence, are the most deleterious. The paradigmatic example is intrafamilial sexual abuse, which is repeated with the inexorable denial of the seriousness of what has been produced. There is a triple disruptive effect: incest itself, perceptual disqualification (this is not bad), and orphanhood as a consequence of self-destitution from the symbolic function of parenthood. As highlighted by the creator of this concept, Masud Khan (1963), the immediate effect, which characterizes cumulative trauma, is its silencing, which can last for decades, until it can be resignified, put into words, and, above all, experienced.

What is the status of that which has been lived without being experienced, which is part of the psyche without being represented, which has not been symbolized and could not be subjective?

The psychic apparatus seeks to link erratic anguish, and representation is perhaps the most elaborate way to deactivate it. "In dreams we do not feel horror because we are oppressed by a sphinx, we dream a sphinx to explain the horror we feel," says Borges (1960, p. 779) in "El Hacedor". The psychic apparatus does not admit that the anguish is left floating. Anguish is Pirandellian, as in *Six Characters in Search of Author* (1993) anguish seeks a representation to which to refer as the author of it. It is in this sense that, in the analytic session dealing with traumatic experiences, construction takes on the value of interpretation. That is to say, one does not necessarily seek a construction that possesses a historical truth, but one that fulfills a function in the dynamics of the psychic apparatus. And Freud (1937) even suggests that the term "construction" and/or "reconstruction" replace that of "interpretation". Viderman (1970) proposes finding a meaning that was absent.

It is less about giving disruptive scenes, impossible to determine in their perceptual conformation, an interpretative value, than about listening to pain while waiting for a suffering that the subject can finally experience—that the subject appropriates the floating statement and that he makes it his own, as a lived enunciation.

The discourse of trauma, says Françoise Davoine (1998), is always carried by someone desubjectivized from the knowledge inscribed in the body, to such an extent that it suspends both the judgment of attribution and the judgment of existence. If time is stopped, it is because for there to be time, it is necessary that there be a subject, and for there to be a subject and therefore repression, a succession of signifiers is necessary. In the case of trauma, the chain of signifiers is interrupted, a hole is produced, and it is precisely then that time stops, waiting for a new signifier. *"Trou-matisme"* (a neologism that plays with *"trou"* = hole), said Lacan (1974). With the contributions of physics, theorized by Albert Einstein and taken up by astrophysics, it can be compared as an analogy with "black holes." According to the Chilean observatory that contributed to obtaining the first image of this hole, black holes are extraordinary cosmic objects, characterized by having an enormous mass in a very compact size. The presence of these objects affects their environment in extreme ways, bending space-time and superheating all surrounding material. Now, how do these black holes act? They are bodies with a lot of mass and little volume, which attracts everything with an immeasurable gravity, to such an extent that not even light can escape their attraction. From the disruptive point of view, it could be said that the potentially traumatic, encysted hole stops time and space in an unconscious redoubt whose membrane prevents its contents from entering into circulation with the signifiers of the unconscious. It would be something like a mark, not yet significant, that is put into circulation when the membrane that surrounds it is permeabilized, blocking its gravitational force that sucks all memory inside the black hole. The subject remains aspirated by this gravitational force, de-subjective, waiting for a process of subjectivation that allows them to emerge from this negative gravitational force.

The traumatic experience is sometimes frightening, but sometimes fascinating. The effect is the same: muteness. "Small sorrows are talkative, big ones are mute," said Seneca (Hippolyte, II, 3; quoted by Montaigne, 1580). The person runs the risk of becoming a statement devoid of enunciation. Even in certain cases in which the person can speak compulsively of the traumatic experience, sometimes without shame, their speech is silenced, or, rather, full of empty speech.

In the latter case, the person is stunned, trapped in the seduction or terror of the traumatic experience, not knowing what to do with it. The subject will appear, in the best of cases, when the person can assume the responsibility of doing something different from what they lived, by disidentifying from the traumatic experience.

The mother of a teenager followed in psychotherapy as a result of incest, herself the victim of incest, presents herself to the first interview, and when she greets me, instead of introducing herself by name, she tells me: "I am the incested woman." The traumatic experience became her identity presentation, instead of declining her identity with her own name. She "was" this statement. The damage suffered is installed as a paradoxical cystic core of an identity emptied of subjectivity. The person "is" the traumatic experience suffered. The person becomes the negative of his true subjectivity and oscillates between a suffocated silence and the scream of Munch, without finding the words that tear the suffering from the interstices of their being.

In the transferential relationship of patients who suffered traumatic experiences, it is particularly convenient to be attentive to all the semiotics of the figural, in particular to the intonations of discourse, through which the unrepresented can be accessed—the changing sound of the voice as a sonorous figural of the vacillations of the lagoon memory of what was lived, but not represented. The voice as a signifier that allows the enunciation of its sound variants to become a word loaded with affection allows us to move from a certain affective aphasia to a discourse subjectivized by emotions that arise as a revitalizing thermal source. Barthes, in *Le plaisir du texte* (1973, p. 43), emphasizes: "What I hide through my language my body says. I can modulate my message, but not my voice."

The voice, its sound, its melody or its disharmony, is the least audible aspect of analytic listening, but at the same time it sometimes allows the affection to be threaded to a possible representation.

From this point of view, I dare to suggest that psychoanalysis, at least in clinical sessions of the traumatic, would be halfway between a conjectural science and a poïesis, in which the subject appears more in the intonation—harmonic or dissonant—of the drive scansion of their voice, in their prosody, rather than in the immobile meaning of an emotionally petrified statement. The word becomes full to the extent that it manages to free the concomitant affection of its confinement.

Only the appearance of a subject who can finally experience their suffering would make it possible, in the words of Paul Valéry (p. 430), that "the past has a future", avoiding the compulsion to deadly repetition or a psychosomatic illness. In that sense, it is not, of course, a question of changing the facts of a traumatic past. Borges (1949), that great clinician of the human soul, said in "The Aleph": "to modify the past is not to modify a single fact; it is to nullify its consequences, which tend to be infinite" (p. 455).

References

Barthes, R. (1973). *Le plaisir du texte*. Paris: Seuil.

Benyakar, M., & Lezica, A. (2005). *Lo traumático*. Buenos: AiresBiblos.

Borges, J. (1949). El Aleph. In: *Obras Completas* (pp. 533–629). Buenos Aires: Emecé, 1974.

Borges, J. (1960). El hacedor. Ragnarok. In: *Obras Completas* (pp. 779–854). Buenos Aires: Emecé, 1974.

Davoine, F. (1998). *The Analytical Discourse of Trauma*. Seminar [not recorded] held at the Ministry of Health, Directorate of Mental Health, Province of Buenos Aires, Argentina.

Duras, M. (1964). *Le ravissement de Lol V. Stein*. Paris: Gallimard.

Freud, S. (1937). Constructiones in analysis. *Standard Edition, Vol. 23*. London: Hogarth Press.

Freud, S. (1950 [1892–1899]). Extracts from the Fliess Papers. In: *Standard Edition, Vol. 1*. London: Hogarth Press, 1966.

Freud, S. (1950 [1895]). Project for a scientific psychology. In: *Standard Edition, Vol. 1*. London: Hogarth Press, 1966.

Khan, M. R. (1963). The concept of cumulative trauma. *Psychoanalytic Study of the Child, 18*: 286–306.

Lacan, J. (1974). *Seminaire 21. Les non-dupes errent. Lesson of February 19*. Unpublished.

Montaigne, M. de (1580). *Les Essais*. Arlès, 1992.

Pirandello, L. (1993). *Sei personaggi in cerca d'autore* [Six characters in search of an author]. Milano: Tascabili Newton.

Quignard, P. (1998). *Vie secrete*. Paris: Gallimard.

Valéry, P. (1942). *Poésies* Paris: Gallimard.

Viderman, S. (1970). *La construction de l'espace analytique*. Paris: Denoël.

17 Viability of psychic change

Between the disruptive of life and the inertia of the deadly, or how to generate fertile psychic changes*

To be alive psychically is to be desiring and to have the elasticity of being able to change—as Freud proposed, to have the capacity to love and work. From time to time, we propose changes, make projects, and wonder if this will be the year or the moment from which we want something to change. Projects can be modest or grandiose. Groucho Marx, with the fine irony that characterized him, said that he had tried to change the world and finally limited himself to changing his tie. What change to achieve when you hardly ever wear a tie any more? What to change? Where do we start? First of all, it is convenient to be clear whether the change is something that one wants for oneself or whether the pressure of change comes from outside—call that "outside" partner, parents, children, boss, religion—or whether, on the contrary, it is an inner force.

The success of a change begins when it is a desire of one's own or, if the proposal comes from the environment, that the person makes it their own. No one changes for the other, although sometimes, in life, there are fruitful encounters that generate questioning, or external events in the surrounding world—accidents, violence, forced migrations, wars—that have a disruptive effect on the psyche and force us to try to elaborate it so that it does not become traumatic. The reasons for the desire for change can be very variable: to stop smoking or quit any addiction, to change partners, jobs, or cities. But, first and foremost, change is a change within oneself. It is not easy to change, we already know that. A human being does not necessarily learn from experience, being the only living being who stumbles at least twice on the same stone. Why, then, is it so difficult to change, beyond the purposes that each one makes to achieve it?

It is because within the human psyche there are opposing forces in permanent struggle, which oppose any modification: life drives (that bind, that unite), death drives (that detach, disunite). The psyche has to

---

* Conference within the framework of the "Night of Ideas", a cycle organized by l'Institut Français and the Embassy of France in Argentina, in 2020: Ostende, January 29 and 30; Mar del Plata, January 31 and February 1

DOI: 10.4324/9781032647791-21

struggle with a certain inertia, in which it is as if it were saying to itself: better the devil you know than the devil you don't. The human psyche is very conservative, it fears the new, it fears surprise, and it fears any modification of a known state, even when that way of functioning causes us problems—sometimes even symptoms and pain. However, the desire for change can become imperative, almost like a way of survival, away from the deadly status quo of the stagnation of more of the same.

In my clinical practice there have been people who told me that they preferred to have a physical illness that allows them to continue in the same vein, without the urgency of change... instead of confronting the psychic work required by producing a change in life. I remember a person who, faced with a state of decay, had to make a differential diagnosis between depression and hypothyroidism. When she brought me the normal results of her thyroid functioning, she told me with some regret: I would have preferred it to be thyroid.... A little thyroid hormone would have been enough. This is also not true, because our psyche can also impact the body, awakening somatizations. Many unhappy marriages endure over time because of the fear of the uncertainty of change, which, in the absence of a certainty of being better, paralyzes and inhibits any attempt at modification. Sometimes the certainty of the inert is preferred to the uncertainty of life. There is no change without some mourning—at least, the mourning of the previous state—there is no change without suffering, a necessary tribute to pay in order to feel better. This change can be done alone or with help. Help can come from someone close emotionally, or with the help of a professional. But to initiate a dynamic of change requires, on the one hand, being convinced of the desire to change, and, on the other hand, recognition of the fragility of each one in the face of the effort that requires being different. In Quino's comic strip (2019), *Mafalda*, we find one of his famous characters, Felipito, grief-stricken and immersed in the following reflections at the beginning of the school term:

> Every time classes start, I get this same thing here! (Putting his hand to his chest). What if I went to a psychoanalyst?—Could a psychoanalyst take away the anguish of going back to school? Would a psychoanalyst get me, Felipe, to go to school happy?—Would a psychoanalyst succeed in transforming me into such a disgusting being?

Behind every request for psychic change persists the opposing forces of non-change, always active and contemporary with the authentic desire for psychic change. Felipito suggests to us, with his reflection on the abject being he would become if he were to change, a true methodology for studying change that is similar to Freud's. Like Felipito, early on he moved away from the monist conception of Jung, who believed that the phenomena of change of the psychic apparatus were the unique expression of a natural dynamism. Although a theory of change is implicit and found in filigree throughout his work, what seems to have polarized Freud the most is the study of resistance to change. It is evident that change costs everyone. They are the unconscious resistances to change, always active, that lurk and hinder the best purposes.

The transformation that psychoanalysis seeks is not a simple adaptation of the person to the environment, as advocated by some schools of psychology and as Felipito feared. Change is not about adapting to the established environment: it consists of a profound change in subjectivity, in letting unconscious desire emerge. Then it will be seen whether or not this change adapts to the established. Sometimes change can be misleading. Not every change is a real change. One can spend years gestating apparent forms of change, which are actually disguises of it. *"Plus ça change, plus c'est la même chose"* (the more it changes, the more it is of the same) says a French proverb, referring to mirages of apparent changes. The process of change must, in order to be authentic, break the previous balance and have a force capable of counterbalancing the forces that sustain the defensive counter investitures. The transformation that psychoanalysis seeks is not a simple adaptation of the person to the environment, as advocated by some schools of psychology and as Felipito feared. Change is not about adapting to the established environment: it consists of a profound change in subjectivity, in letting unconscious desire emerge. Then it will be seen whether or not this change adapts to the established. There is no change without deligation, without a departure from the usual ways of functioning.

Guiseppe Tomasi di Lampedusa, in *The Gattopardo* (1957), has Tancredo, a young, acerbic Sicilian nobleman enlisted, apparently against the interests of his class, in Garibaldi's armies that promoted the unification of Italy, say: "If we want everything to remain as it is, everything needs to change" (p. 47). Is this just political cynicism, or deep knowledge of the conservative function of the human psyche?

Freud explains that the patient defends himself energetically against the suppression of symptoms and the restoration of the usual mode of his psychic processes, as the forces that oppose the change of the morbid state are the same as those that, at a given moment, had provoked that state. How to get out of this "impasse"? Psychoanalytic treatment sometimes gestates in the psychic structure of the patient a certain disorder, a relative chaos, which can arouse fears. Thus, some parents who consult for a depressed child tend to worry when they become more turbulent when the child comes out of their depression. Beyond the fact that the previous order is achieved to the detriment of the creative capacity of the person, every modification is experienced as a disorder, as a cause of restlessness, distrust, perhaps a form of evil.

Alberto Rojo (2013), a specialist in quantum physics, recalls that we create a new skin every two weeks, a liver every year and a half, and our skeleton is renewed every ten years (p. 57). It is still debated what happens to neurons, but it is known that in the face of brain damage, new neural connections are generated. The gut microbiotic changes all the time. Without talking about aging or pathology, our body changes without us doing anything. And our psyche: are we the same at the end of life? Does the self exist? Does monolithic identity exist? Or are we different versions of ourselves simultaneously and successively? *"Je suis un autre"* [I am another], the French poet Rimbaud said (1871, p. 986). The so-called exact sciences have always tried to describe what they call laws of nature: laws of general order that would allow us to predict events and prevent chaos. Disorder had no place, and the notion of chaos enjoyed no prestige among the followers of positivist thought.

For a long time science was Platonic, valuing the mathematical forms that manifested in a purer way the modalities attributed to the great demiurge: purity, superiority, harmony, logical transparency. The Cartesians, in love with harmonies and well-groomed logical processes, traditionally maintained that behind the apparent disorders of nature there is a disguised order. However, contemporary science—meteorology, physics, mathematics—is increasingly interested in the chaotic processes of nature, and a theory of chaos has emerged. Whether they are disordered materials or turbulent processes, chaos is fully recognized as an object of knowledge. The researchers, taking up Poincaré's vocabulary, try to model everything that chaos contains as strange.

Without pretending to extrapolate the growing interest of science in the chaotic processes of nature to the psychic apparatus, one might ask whether a certain degree of chaos is not inherent in every process of psychic change. Too much bonding perhaps prevents chaos but coagulates psychic energy, like inert cement. The fear of living with a certain degree of chaos petrifies the psyche. The person clings to the known, to the deadly, pretending to avoid a certain internal disorder. But to achieve a creative psychic change, you can't avoid being crossed by the fear of processes of disengagement. I find it useful to think that for change to actually take place, it is necessary to have the ability to accept a certain degree of mobilizing psychic chaos.

I understand, by mobilizing psychic chaos, the acceptance within the psychic apparatus of a certain amount of disengagement, of a circulation of free psychic energy, without seeking to unite it hastily in a new representation, to the acceptance of a certain degree of disintrication of the life and death drives and to a relative independence of the latter—that is, accepting that something dies in order to live again. This requires admitting that the interior closet can be disordered for a while. Many people are distressed by not feeling "normal" (assuming that normality exists...), but there is a certain form of "normality," coagulated, viscous, which, rather than normality, I would call *"normopathy"*—that is, a rigid and unimaginative search for a pretended normalized normality, according to icons and social prejudices, bordering on the pathological. In that case the person could say to himself: I am no longer myself; I am the one I suppose they expect me to be (my environment, society)—a form of alienation that attacks subjectivity.

The fear of living with a certain degree of chaos petrifies psychic instances. The confrontation with pain, sometimes with failure, with depression and the deepest hopelessness, with those moments when everything seems to disintegrate, is often the first step to the creative act of the artist or to a renewed energy and pleasure in living. Overcoming this resistance implies accepting death in oneself, as Hegel would say—elaborate the paradox of death accepted in itself as a condition for remaining psychically alive. Patients growing interest in their own dreams (in which they contact their unconscious desire) and their renewed capacity for humor (which generates pleasure) seem to me two privileged axes to evaluate the possibility of change. Speaking of humor, I will end my text with a quote from the cartoonist Tute. In one of his drawings, we see a person lying on the couch of an analyst to whom he says the following: "I want me to do well... but I don't know what my unconscious thinks." *Last but not least*, it does not hurt to remember Nietzsche (1883), a suggestion that seems to me extremely hopeful of the desire for change beyond the fear it may unleash: "You must have chaos within you to give birth to a dancing star" (p. 59).

References

Lampedusa, G. T. di (1957). *El Gattopardo* [The leopard]. Buenos Aires: Losada, 2004.

Nietzsche, F. (1883). *Así habló Zaratustra* [Thus Spake Zarathustra]. Madrid: Alianza, 2011.

Quino (2019). *Mafalda. Colección completa, Vols 1–10.* Buenos Aires: Ediciones de la Flor.

Rojo, A. (2019). *Borges y la física cuántica* [Borges and quantum physics]. Buenos Aires: Siglo Veintiuno.

Rimbaud, A. (1871). Lettres du voyant. In: Œuvres completes. Paris: Gallimard, 2009.

18 What hurts you?

Psychic vulnerability and somatic disorder*

Aphaniosis is the name I will give to this adult patient, who came to my office referred by his clinician. Two years had elapsed since the date of referral and his request for an interview. He did not understand, he tells me, why his doctor proposed an interview with a psychoanalyst, when in reality (the word reality will be a recurring word in his lexicon) he had no psychological problems. He did admit to having some somatic problems, which were difficult to solve: basically, ulcerative colitis and uncontrollable essential hypertension. Regarding complex reaction to drugs, he used to express secondary reactions to them, which motivated the interruption and change of medication. Describing the infinity of medicaments he was taking would be almost equivalent to revealing his identity, to such an extent did they define him in his uniqueness.

Aphaniosis put his scientific training at the service of his paranoid personality, which sought—needless to say, fruitlessly—to control circumstances and his body. He methodically took his blood pressure four times a day, data that he graphed daily in great detail in curves. The values were erratic, without being able to justify the variations by forgetting to take some medication, which never happened. The addition of anxiolytics to his treatment plan allowed him to decrease beta-blockers and diuretics, without us being able to explain the regular increase in his blood pressure on Sunday nights. He did not know, given the proximity of the beginning of the work week, whether this was the result of a phobia of his work, which carried enormous responsibility, or the consequence of a friendly weekend spent with his family.

Aphaniosis not only did not express any desires, it was impossible for him to categorize his emotions. He didn't know what anguish was, he didn't know what grief meant, nor sadness, nor anger: maintaining great self-control, the only thing that escaped his control were the tension figures and bloody diarrhea. Alexithymia—that is, the inability to qualify

* A shorter version of this text was presented at the XXIII Argentine Congress of Psychiatry of the APSA (Association of Argentine Psychiatrists), Mar del Plata, April 19–21, 2007.

DOI: 10.4324/9781032647791-22

their emotions—is one of the characteristics described in patients with somatic expression of their psychic pathology.

Aphaniosis did not express conflicts or psychic pain: only his body spoke, but as an exteriority, as a voice-over, almost as a foreign body that had nothing to do with his self. He talked to me about his body the way someone who describes the damage to his car's engine to a mechanic. He was not hurt by the psychic expression of his unconscious conflicts in the form of anguish, but by his large intestine hurt in the form of colic. His body, lived as persecutory, did not allow him to forget that when someone tries to deny the psychic expression of conflicts and their consequent psychic pain, it is the body that becomes a paradigmatic sign of a complex semiotics to decipher. Paraphrasing Roland Barthes (1970), I will say that interpreting a somatic symptom is not giving it a meaning (better or worse founded): on the contrary, it is appreciating what plural it is made of.

In the symptom of conversion disorder, the body is, for the hysteric, an instrument of symbolization. For the psychosomatic patient the body is a victim. If the first sends a message and speaks to his body, the second suffers in his body with an obscured, denied message. Alexander (1987), following the tradition of the Chicago School in the 1950s, included among the so-called psychosomatic diseases the famous seven (the holy seven), like the plagues of Egypt: gastro-duodenal ulcer, ulcer hemorrhagic recto colitis, essential hypertension, rheumatoid arthritis, thyrotoxicosis, bronchial asthma, and neurodermatitis. Each of these diseases was associated with a characterological personality type—in other words, certain characteristics of the personality were considered to predict the somatic symptomatology by establishing a linear causal relationship.

Personally, I feel much closer to the psychosomatic school in Paris, whose mentor has been Pierre Marty (1992). The school does not associate personality with symptomatology, but describes a certain type of psychic functioning that predisposes to somatic symptomatology, without predicting or establishing a causal relationship. For this school, somatic symptomatology covers the entire pathology of body expression, by proposing the uniqueness of somatopsychic functioning. It is not possible to predict which will be the effector organ of somatic pathology, this will depend on multiple factors, including genetics, diet, and environment. But it will be possible to predict the increased risk of expression of the pathology through the body.

Already in 1911, Walter B. Cannon, the physiologist, had demonstrated the physiological effects of emotions that influence the whole organism through the cortico–hypothalamic–pituitary axis involved in the regulation of homeostasis of the internal environment (Cannon, 1915). Since then, numerous studies have shown, for example, the influence of depression on the lowering of immune defenses, with the increased risk of the expression of chronic diseases, which are sometimes reversible and sometimes irreversible. It is not uncommon for cancer to develop during grief.

Lately, the increase in C-reactive protein in cases of depression has been highlighted as an increased risk of generating a cardiovascular accident, even in the absence of other concomitant risk factors, such as smoking, increased cholesterol or diabetes.

Psychoanalysis made it possible to establish the psychodynamic principles that govern and organize the psychosomatic unity of a person. Duality disappears. The human being is psychosomatic by definition. Substantified, as a noun, it defines a field of study. Applied as an adjective, "psychosomatically," it is redundant. In that sense I propose to abandon the denomination of psychosomatic as an adjective and to replace it with pathologies of expression to somatic predominance, the latter intervening, when the psyche fails to function, as a barrier of containment of conflicts. Somatic pathology appears when the psyche becomes vulnerable and fails to contain conflicts within it. It is not uncommon in the clinical session to hear patients say that they feel relieved at the diagnosis of cancer.

For Moty Benyakar (2019), what our neurovegetative system does is to transform factual presentation into mental elaboration. It will be after of the transformation of the factual into the mental that it will reach the level of the psyche. Not every mental process reaches the level of the psyche. It is thought that if it is mental, it is because it is conscious. The conscious and the unconscious are psychic and non-mental processes. Those processes that are elaborated from the neurovegetative we will call mentalized processes, and those that acquire the psychic dimension processes of the psyche. That which comes from the factual and impacts the person we will call mentalized processes; those that pass from the mentalized to the psychic will be called somatopsychic processes; and those that pass from the psychic to the somatic will be called somatizing processes, says Moty Benyakar.

Recently, a patient whose symptoms required the differential diagnosis between depression and hypothyroidism was heartbroken by the normal results of thyroid function... adding: "I would have paid for something to be found in my thyroid that explained what I am experiencing..." Beyond these extreme cases, we have all known the "well-being" of having "achieved" a flu or a low back pain that allows us to regressively stay in bed, leaving suspended for a few days the conflicts that we could not solve. They constitute transient overflows of the psychic apparatus, without serious consequences. The soma operates, as well as an offer of truce to the unspeakable opposing forces that are undecided in our unconscious: the soma, as a defensive mechanism of the self.

In general, the somatic response can be functional, as in some headaches, or lesions, as in ulcers. Psychosomatic disorganization can be reversible or, in some cases, irreversible, leading the patient to a terminal illness. What characterizes the psychic functioning of people at increased risk of somatization? The Psychosomatic School of Paris describes several psychic mechanisms that move away from classical nosography and are closer to the pathologies of emptiness, described by André Green (1990). From the metapsychological point of view, the economic point of view prevails. Its Freudian antecedent would be the current neuroses, although the symptom is not shown so much as a neurotic screen, but as a translation in the body of a difficulty in thinking and for a verbal expression of conflicts—as an overflow of the capacity of the psychic apparatus to contain and elaborate conflicts.

There is, in the first place, operative thought or operative life, as Marty (1992) later called it: it is a conscious thought, without connection with imaginary representative movements and with little fantastic capacity. It does not use classical neurotic or psychotic mechanisms. It is a thought devoid of libidSmadjao that tends to deny aggressiveness and avoids psychic investitures. The associations that the patient brings are, when they exist at all, poor or repetitive. The current and the factual acquire an overvaluation. The claudication of the imaginary world and dream life, together with the expressive lack of affections and the over-investiture of secondary processes, to the detriment of primary processes, is very degraded. This impacts on the scarcity or harshness of dream life. There is something like gaps in the preconscious, which loses its potential as a mediator between the unconscious and consciousness, losing its porosity and becoming something like a dam without gates. The richer the preconscious is shown in representations linked to each other, the more the eventual pathology tends to be located in a mental aspect. It is in this sense that Marty considers the preconscious as the revolving door of psychosomatic economics.

Secondly there is what Marty called the essential depression. They are depressions without purpose or self-accusation, or conscious guilt, in which the feelings of devaluation and narcissistic wounding are oriented towards the somatic sphere. There is no experience of sadness. The person complains of tiredness and apathy. They usually consume vitamin complexes and magnesium salts; there is like a call to the body to speak, a consequence of failures in the psychic processing of emotional experiences. They deny anguish, including signal distress, which is, as is well known, protective of the organism. It is as if the subject's ability to protect themselves from the risk to come was lost, or perhaps never reached. Desires have disappeared, to make way for stereotyped interests or a mere demand for the satisfaction of needs. The unconscious does not emit signals; it remains overshadowed by a prevalence of the factual. The death instinct prevails. (Note that Marty speaks here of instinct and not of drive, insofar as the drive includes representation, which is absent in essential depression. Instinct is not translated as drive and its psychic representative, but would pass directly to the body, without psychic representation.) The existence of desires is searched for in vain, and only automatic interests are found. The absence of communication with the unconscious constitutes a true rupture of its own history.

Thirdly, there is progressive disorganization, which corresponds in Freudian terms to a de-intricating of the drives, with a predominance of the detachment of the death drive. There is a regressive movement that does not find a limit, as in fertile regression. There are no regressive arrests. For Marty, there would be a drive monism: without libido, the death instinct reigns, which to the extent that it reigns for a prolonged time without libidinal reorganizations, can lead to real death. The ideal Self occupies an excessive, deadly place, a place without subtleties, of great rigidity and cruelty, incompatible with a post-oedipal superego. It leaves no room for intimate deliberations or transitory regressions (how to return here from primary narcissism, other than by dying?). It differs from regressive disorganization, which is limited in time and always rich in reorganizing potential. It is a body resource that stabilizes homeostasis—regression to soma as a libidinal resource.

Psychic regressive mechanisms are combined with somatic, counter evolutionary regressive mechanisms—for example, when angina or back pain "forces and allows" us, simultaneously, to make a stop in the maelstrom of constant activity, as a way to avoid thinking. In a neurotic structure, angina or back pain may allow you to reconnect with your own thoughts, which had been set aside by alienating hyperactivity. In the course of life, the psychosomatic balance can be temporarily altered by exhaustion of psychic resources, with the appearance of circumstantial somatic symptoms that try to establish a parenthesis before the overload and daily tensional demand. There is then a momentary disorganization to certain points of fixation, due to lack of psychosomatic integration, but with good levels of reorganization and recovery of lost balance. In other cases, the somatic manifestation is a useful alarm signal to promote changes in the attitude to life. In progressive disorganization, on the other hand, the regressive movement is not stopped by any valid regressive organization; the fixation does not function as a barrier, which can lead to irreversible disorganization processes. Certain hyperactivities constitute true behaviors of exhaustion. They are attempts to generate an evacuation of an excess of non-metaphorical psychic load: what Claude Smadja calls self-calming processes.[1] This difficulty in processing the excessive aspect of psychic loads is the essence of somatization processes, according to Marty. He calls it a pure charge of excitement, which does not acquire impulsive value, to the extent that it does not process through the psychic representative of the drive. It discharges directly into the organ, without a psychic representative.

According to this scheme, a good mentalization gives rise to a reversible disease—regardless of the classical psychoanalytic nosography—while difficulty in mentalizing conflicts gives rise to evolutionary processes. The sequence is that a more or less profound disorganization of psychic functioning is followed by somatization. Quoting Pessoa (2002), I will say that the psychosomatic patient "dominates his emotions, but not his feelings." The discharge short-circuits the psyche and directly hits the body. A good mindset deals with the quantity and quality of representations of a given individual. It includes the three fundamental qualities of the preconscious: (1) thickness of the set of representative formations; (2) fluidity of the links between the representations; (3) permanence of functioning without progressive disorganization.

In progressive disorganizations, word representations can be reduced to representations of things, losing most of the affective, symbolic, metaphorical components acquired during development, or eventually never acquired. It is as if there were no representations of words with their symbolic potentiality, but merely representations of thing. In his novel, *Gulliver's Travels*, Jonathan Swift (1726, p. 366) imagines a conversation in a language in which there are no words but, instead, things to replace them. Thus, each person would be required to travel with countless things, to such an extent that such artificial conversation would require "carrying on his back a great array of things, unless he can afford one or two sturdy servants to assist him. I have seen many times, two of these wise men, almost overwhelmed by the weight of their burdens" (p. 366). For my part, I imagine that, in the case of psychosomatic illnesses, each person carries a heavy backpack of representation-things, which bend his back and make his body groan.

In Marty's work (1992), instinct and drive coexist. Instinct would be pure energetic charge without representation that directly impacts the soma. The drive, although Freud places it on the border between the somatic and the psychic, cannot be known except through its representatives—that is, the affectionate representative and the representative-representation of the drive. For Marty, both are absent or scarce in the case of psychosomatic patients, leaving a symbolic gap that causes instinct to strike directly.

In this type of patient, drug treatments should be given according to a delicate alchemy. Doses that are too low do not give the body the opportunity to rediscover a homeostasis that allows the previous biological defenses to be reinvigorated. Those that are too many or too strong decapitate the symptom by preventing the person from questioning their own wavering subjectivity. As we said with Santiago Kovadloff in an article a few years ago:

> the apparent therapeutic triumph consists then in imposing a pharmacological order where the symptoms are only conceived as an expression of chaos, without any fruitful metaphorical relief. It thus works in mirror, that is, slavishly, with respect to an accelerated society that demands immediate responses, without taking into account temporality, that is, searching, waiting and processes.

The great excluded from the system is the person. We are confronted in this way with a logic that speaks in the third person: the symptom, the drug, the pharmacological monitoring and the diagnosis by images. There is a risk of a surrender of the physician's subjectivity, of the transferential relationship and a neutralization of the patient as a subject. The clinic runs the risk of becoming disinterested in the meaning that the symptom has for each person affected by it, moving away from it as an irredeemable value, favouring the patient's aliena-tion from his own subjectivity." [Kovadloff & Tesone, 2002]

Joyce McDougall (1989) even speaks of psychosomatosis to highlight the aspect of current substitute psychosis in some somatosis, hence the fear of "madness" if they abandon the somatic symptoms to which they cling. If the body becomes persecutory, the unconscious becomes even more so. Somatic symptoms can be the displacement in the body of an excruciating mental pain, desperate attempt at self-healing. Therefore, when attempt-ing a psychic approach to the patient's problem, the therapist will face a tenacious resistance to abandon somatic symptoms whose disappearance, paradoxically, is feared. They are patients who, the more symptoms in the body they present, the more they achieve a deceptive peace in their psy-che. Words are reduced to the state of things.

It is the analyst's job to find missing links, or even to create them. The approach of a psychosomatic patient will not be the same as of a neurotic patient. The lifting of repression, childhood amnesia, and interpretation do not acquire the same value as in neurosis. Given the associative inabil-ity of the patient, the absence of representations available in their own pre-conscious, the analyst must do something like "lend their preconscious," finding the metaphorical meaning of the symptom, as they will not be able to resort to a traditional scheme for the cure in which they expect the patient to associate freely. Here, the patient feels free not to associate. The therapy will be face-to-face, the purely verbal is less likely to be used, and sensory-perceptual mechanisms are alluded to. A psychic—even pathological—reorganization is sought more than the urgency of resolv-ing conflicts.

For André Green (1990), it is convenient to consider borderline cases, and patients with somatic expression are, to a large extent, borderline cases of analyzability. In such cases it is necessary to offer the patient a double proposal: to give containment to its contents and to give content to its containment. The therapeutic framework thus acquires the value of reducing extreme stresses through the mental apparatus of the analyst. The analytic technique of neuroses is deductive, that of limit cases, from countertransference. Hence its greater randomness. In these cases of the dual role of the analyst, as interpreter and object-support of the transfer-ence, the second is the most important.

It would seem useful for the patient—and in addition to health systems—to include in periodic clinical check-ups, a predictive assessment of the risks of somatosis of patients, according to their psychic psychodynamics, perhaps in collaboration with specialized teams.

To conclude my speech, but without pretending to conclude, I propose that, since neurosis protects from somatization, we live our neuroses thoroughly, let a certain tenor of anguish emerge, admit despite ourselves some perverse trait or some well-known psychotic nucleus, and be as happy as possible—without forgetting that, as Emil Cioran (1987) said, "those who feel good are not real. They have everything but being—which confers improbable health." And then he adds: "Getting out of life unscathed—it could happen, but in reality, it never happens."

Note

1 The self-soothing procedures of the ego in the adult refer to the failure of the organization of secondary auto-eroticism and of the functions of representation and phantasy. "These are activities that seek to master a state of tension of internal excitement, when the psychic means of ligation are lacking." The subject resorts to motor skills and perceptuality, in a contradiction, because at the same time they are calming and exciting which makes them repetitive to the point of exhaustion.

References

Alexander, F. (1987). *Psychosomatic Medicine: Its Principles and Applications* (2nd ed.). New York: Norton.

Barthes, R. (1970). *S/Z*. París: Seuil.

Benyakar, M. (2019). *Mental, Psyche, the Introduct and Memory*. Personal comunication.

Cannon, W. B. (1915). Bodily changes. In: *Pain, Hunger, Fear and Rage*. New York: Appleton.

Cioran, E. (1987). *Aveux et anathèmes*. París: Gallimard.

Green, A. (1990). *La folie privée, psychanalyse des cas-limites*. Paris: Gallimard.

Kovadloff, S., & Tesone, J. E. (2002). La psiquiatría se aleja del hombre [Diary]. *La Nación* (Buenos Aires), 1 October.

Marty, P. (1992). *La psychosomatique de l'adulte*. París: PUF.

McDougall, J. (1989). Théâtres du corps. In: *Le psychosoma en psychanalyse*. Paris: Gallimard.

Pessoa, F. (with Soares, B.) (2002). *El libro del desasosiego*. Buenos Aires: Emecé.

Smadja, C. (1993). Les procédés autocalmants du Moi. *Revue Française de Psychosomatique*, 4: 11.

Swift, J. (1726). *Los viajes de Gulliver* [Gulliver's travels]. Buenos Aires: Luarna.

19 Transformations of the formless

Painting and psychoanalysis*

It was spherical mirrors that gave rise to Lacan's (1949) later theorization of the mirror stage and the deceptive Self of the Imaginary. What you see is not necessarily the thing, but you also don't know exactly what you hear—and even less if one takes into account that perceptions are not the thing and that the image of the thing or the word that is heard enters into an associative framework in the psychic apparatus of the person. It then links it to other perceptions, sensations, fantasies, memories, and previous psychic strata, in continuous reformulation, which means that the perception is not given by the thing, but by the singularity of the subject. Scopophilia and the pleasure of looking, voyeurism, also allows me the neologism of "listening" or the pleasure of listening. The perception is modified by desire. Painting is a visual art that appeals mainly to the gaze of generally framed images.

Psychoanalysis apparently appeals to listening to a discourse within another type of framework, the setting of the session, but which also serves to frame, according to psychoanalytic rules, the encounter between analyst and analysand. It appeals to senses that seem to diverge, but are closer than it seems. If painting and psychoanalysis have something in common, it is the need that both have figuration. This is evident with sleep theory. The manifest content of the dream has been an inspiration for numerous painters. I do not intend to make an exhaustive study of these works, but let us say that in medieval and Renaissance iconography, representing the dream meant, above all, representing, isolating, the fantastic content within an illuminated frame of a particular diffuse and continuous light. Examples of this are Piero della Francesca's *The Dream of Constantine* and Vittore Carpaccio's *The Dream of St. Ursula*.

Vittorio Fagone (1991) points out that, in modern art, romantic passion visits the dream without isolating it, as a place of great communicative symbols, obsessions, and projective catharsis. Among Francisco Goya's,

* Published in *Calibán, Journal of the Latin American Federation of Psychoanalysis (Fepal)*, Vol. 16, No. 1, 2018.

DOI: 10.4324/9781032647791-23

we find, for example, *The Author Dreaming* and a series of ink drawings gathered under the title of *Dreams*. For Goya, who goes beyond the thought of the Enlightenment, sleep, more than reason, reveals the nature of things. The great merit of Goya, highlighted by Baudelaire (1975) consists in creating the plausible monster: it is impossible to differentiate the suture line, the point of union between the real and the fantastic; it is a vague boundary that the most subtle analyst could not draw, and each piece of art is transcendent and natural at the same time. Their monsters were born viable, harmonic. No one dared more than he did to explore absurdity. It is what art makes of the "natural" and creating new ways of life.

Influenced by Freud, with the *Cadavres exquis* of the Surrealists, a series of words or images made by multiple hands between the years 1920 and 1930 are grouped together. André Breton and his friends, with automatic writing, then drawings, tried to make a production of the collective unconscious. We see how writing and image, but also spontaneous discourse from a group playful perspective, are intimately related. Now, returning to the psychoanalytic method: does the perception of the discourse of the analysis consist only of listening; is it the auditory and not the visual that enters the analyst's consciousness? In my opinion, nothing is less likely.

In *On Aphasia: A Critical Study* (1891), Freud speaks for the first time of language apparatus; emphasizing the difference between word representation (linked to the preconscious) and thing representation (linked to the unconscious). To the representation of words, he assigns four components: the sound image, the visual image of the letter, the motor image of the language, and the motor image of the reading. And he then concludes that the word is a complex representation composed of the aforementioned images—that is, that the word corresponds to a complicated associative process where the enumerated elements of visual, acoustic, and kinetic origin enter into conjunction with each other. Later he emphasizes that it is impossible to separate representation and association, we cannot have any sensation without associating it immediately.

If thinking in pictures is imperfect thinking, thinking in words pretends to forget that consciousness needs to see in order to conceive (Khan, 2001). There is an apparent heterogeneity between word and image. Do I dare to say that there is no listening to the discourse—that is, the auditory—without immediately the auditory image, as Freud calls it, not being immediately associated with other images, be they olfactory, visual, or kinetic. All perception enters into an associative reticulation of images. Everything that is presented to the analyst's listening will have to be figurative, moving from the unrepresented (as in the remembrance of neurotics) or the unrepresentable (in the pathology of trauma) to the representable and then represented in a possible symbolization

Green (2001) proposes a plural significance of figurability: the relationship with the visual would be nothing but a particular, rich, but not exclusive aspect. Diderot (1964) wondered: And it was answered: forms... and what else? ... Forms; I don't know the thing. That the image of the thing is not the thing was immortalized in René Magritte's famous painting of the pipe, in which a pipe is seen... with the inscription: *"Ceci n'est pas une pipe"* [this is not a pipe], since what we see is its image. The plasticity of the visual is subject to how our memory, our associative reticulate, falsifies perception under the effect of desire. Perceived forms are expressions produced by recomposition of previously perceived forms that lend themselves to substitution operations in an infinite metonymy. Such substitutions do not differentiate between visual images, acoustic images, or olfactory or kinetic images.

The word, in the form of enunciation, which is produced by a given subject, is heard as a representation by the analyst, and this representation is not merely acoustic, it includes the entire perceptual reticulation of the analyst, in which the visual does not remain excluded. The prototype of each representation is mostly visual, even for non-visual art. I add to the representation the prosody of the discourse, which is like a palette of colors, which listens and represents the rhythm and not only the meaning of the enunciated: what Barthes (1981) called the grain of the voice in the semiotics of listening. The listening of the discourse of patient by the analyst is an exteriority that promotes the deepest interior of the analyst An exteriority that becomes an interiority, in a sharing of intimacy in an asymmetrical way, but entertained by a singular space that promotes at the same time as the intimacy of saying and representing.

The association called free of the analysis is conjugated by the association, at the same time free and oriented by the discourse of the analysand, in an associative intertwining full of images "heard." As François Jullien (2013, p. 18) suggests, the space of "intimacy that opens up unfolds over them like a tent to stay." Thus, through the intimate, the French philosopher points out, the traditional relationships of inside and outside are broken. The intimacy of the frame keeps associated "withdrawal and sharing," typical of the intimate, where voices and arborescent visual representations circulate in a framework woven by the protagonists of the analytic encounter.

As a result of censorship, we know that dreams are deformations and fragmentations of representations that aim to disguise themselves and mask unconscious desire. The apparent absurdity of the manifest content is due to that cross-dressing that realizes the dream to deceive censorship. With the work of the dream is the whole system of representations that returns to the state of malleable, plastic matter. Unconsciously it includes condensation, displacement, and consideration of figurability. Consciously, upon awakening, a vain attempt to give a logical coherence to the dream will only contribute to disguise it. I insist on the consideration of figurability, since the dream has to represent in images an unconscious desire. To be able to express it in words, the manifest content must be fragmented and develop the associations of the patient. This difficulty in expressing an image, as a painting, emotions, ideas, memories—in short, a whole reticulated at the same time remembrance and affective—resembles what a painter can feel in front of his canvas.

Freud, in the *Interpretation of Dreams* (1900, pp. 312–313), warns that:

> When the whole mass of these dream-thoughts is brought under the pressure of the dream-work, and its elements are turned about, broken into fragments and jammed together-almost like pack-ice, the question arises of what happens to the logical connections which have hitherto formed its frame-work. What representation do dreams provide for "it," "because," "just as," "although," "either," " or," and all the other conjunctions without which we cannot understand sentences or speeches? Dreams disregard all these conjunctions, and they take over and manipulate. The restoration of the connections which the dream-work has destroyed is a task which has to be performed by the interpretative process. The plastic arts of painting and sculpture labor, indeed, under a similar limitation as compared with poetry, which can make use of speech; and here once again the reason for their incapacity lies in the nature of the material which these two forms of art manipulate in their effort to express something. Before painting became acquainted with the laws of expression by which it is governed, it made attempts to get over this handicap. In ancient paintings small labels were hung from the mouth of the persons represented, containing in written characters the speeches which the artist despaired of representing pictorially." And later he adds: "But just as the art of painting eventually found a way of expressing, by means other than the floating labels, at least the intention of the words of the personages represented—affection, threats, warnings, and so on- so too there is a possible means by which dreams can take account of some of the logical relations between their dream thoughts, by making an appropriate modification in the method of representation characteristic of dreams."

If there is one thing in common between psychoanalysis and painting, it is that both are concerned with representations and their destinies and how to shape the report. Paul Klee (1985) says to pick up what rises from the depths to transmit it further, tries to grasp the trace and retain its movement, and concludes that never or nowhere is the form an acquired result. The dream, traversed and interpreted, does not exhaust its significance. There is a point, says Freud, by which he gets lost in the unknowable, which he calls the navel of sleep and opens to the unknown. Would it be something like the equivalent of the vanishing point in painting? The subject goes from the informable to the forms, from the forms to the formation of a representation, in a creative poiesis.

Figuration for psychoanalysts has the advantage of assuming the existence of a background that remains in the shadow of the unconscious. The background is the impulsive. Salomon Resnik (1994) emphasizes that the human being cannot see himself without the presence of another, and when he says the other, he includes the other in himself. The function of the analyst would be to make visible the invisibility of the unconscious. The passage to the visible then generates both fascination and horror. It involves confronting the unexpected, transforming the revealed into perceptible images, putting light in the darkness of the inner night. To represent would be a way of making thought present in the form of images, a certain sensory-perceptual experience that is always relational. Merleau-Ponty (1964) stresses that perception exists only to the extent that someone can perceive it. In that sense the sensible exists only because there are living beings in the universe.

The Italian philosopher Emmanuele Coccia (2010) affirms that language is, first and foremost, one of the forms of existence of the sensible. If we speak, it is because we are particularly sensitive to images. There is no language without image; this is but a form of higher sensitivity. The word, the ear, vision, all our experience is nothing but an operation of multiplication of the real, insofar as it uses images. Living beings do not merely passively receive the sensible, because at the same time they actively produce it. In this the human being surpasses all animals.

In "The Psycho-Analytic View of Psychogenic Disturbance of Vision" (1910), Freud asserts that the hysterical blind see, however, in a certain sense, though not in the full sense. They are blind only to consciousness; in the unconscious they are seers. The hysterical blind is not blind as a result of the self-suggestive representation that they do not see, but by the dissociation between unconscious and conscious processes in the act of seeing. And he adds later, bringing into play the oppositions between psychic instances and the repression of the erotic pleasure of seeing: it is as if, in the individual, a punishing voice is raised that says: "Since you sought to misuse your organ of sight for evil sensual pleasures, it is fitting that you should not see anything at all anymore" (p. 217).

Although Freud wrote this text about hysterical blindness, could not the hypothesis that the subject sees what his superego allows him to see be advanced? Each one of us says and listens to what their psychic instances allow them to run, in a perceptive framework that captures what is perceived and transforms it. Isn't the blind spot of the unconscious at the service of avoiding conflict by escaping from the symptom's vanishing point?

The symbolic representation that unknots the symptom, on the other hand, is waiting for a psychic transformation of the formless into a figurability that allows the elaborative metaphor to be presented. It is very suggestive to conclude provisionally regarding the bond that unites verb and image—that is, what representation can contribute to the discourse in psychoanalysis, as proposed by Jacques Ancet (2013) in one of his poems:

On voit, oui. Mais quoi?	One sees, yes. But what?
Ce qu'on entend.	What one hears.
Comment ça?	How can this be?
Des images dans l'oreille.	Images in the ear.
Dans l'oreille?	In the ear?
Oui, là où parle la voix.	Yes, where the voice is
Et que dit-elle?	speaking.
Ce qu'on voit.	And what does it say?
	What one sees.

References

Ancet, J. (2013). *Portrait d'une ombre & retrato de una sombra* [Bilingual edition], trans. C. Madero. Buenos Aires: Alción.

Barthes, R. (1981). *Le grain de la voix. Entretiens 1962–1980.* París: Seuil.

Baudelaire, Ch. (1975). *Oeuvres complètes.* París: Gallimard.

Coccia, E. (2010). *La vida sensible.* Spanish trans. by M. T. D'Meza. Buenos Aires: Marea, 2011.

Diderot, D. (1964). Éléments de physiologie. París: Honoré Champion, 2004.

Fagone, V. (1991). *Il sognorivela la nature delle cose.* Milan: Mazzotta.

Freud, S. (1891). *On Aphasia: A Critical Study.* New York: International Universities Press, 1953.

Freud, S. (1900). *Interpretations of Dreams (Part 1).* In: *Standard Edition, Vol. 4.* London: Hogarth Press.

Freud, S. (1910). The psycho-analytic view of psychogenic disturbance of vision. In: *Standard Edition, Vol. 11.* London: Hogarth Press.

Green, A. (2001). Que sont les forms? *Revue Française de Psychanalyse,* 65: 1121–1127.

Jullien, F. (2013). *Lo íntimo. Lejos del ruidoso amor,* Spanish trans. by S. Mattoni. Buenos Aires: El Cuenco de Plata, 2016.

Khan, L. (2001). La figurabilité. *Revue Française de Psychanalyse,* 64: 983–1053.

Klee, P. (1985). *Théorie de l'art moderne.* París: Folio-Essais.

Lacan, J. (1949). Le stade du miroir comme formateur de la function du Je telle qu'elle nous est révélée dans l'expérience psychaanalytique. Écrits. Paris: Seuil, 1966.

Merleau-Ponty, M. (1964). *L'Oeil et l'esprit.* París: Gallimard.

Resnik, S. (1994). *La visibilità dell'inconscio.* Venice: Teda Edizioni.

20 Commemorating, remembering, forgetting*

Commemorating

For the Greeks, commemorating was a subtle alchemy between remembering and forgetting. We will take a tour of the traditional value of remembering in psychoanalysis, introducing something perhaps little taken up by theory, such as the hypothesis about the value it acquires in a certain form of forgetting, not that at the service of repression or cleavage, but that is necessary to promote the creative power of memory. The importance that a civilization devotes to memory is measured by the place it occupies and in the practices of memory, either by an individual or in collective commemoration. The past was preserved in Greece through the use of inscriptions and archives. But at first the archives were not written; they were entrusted to the oral memory of certain magistrates or officials; called "mnemons", these were depositories. The Greek language has several terms to designate the monument, the building of remembrance: *mnemata, mnemeia, mnemosuna*. These terms qualify the memory without being limited to the materiality of the building. The memory is materialized as an object or in an act: tombstones, crowns of victory, hymns, ritual feasts. The originality of Greek memory is not given by the exceptional character of its monuments but, on the contrary, by having dematerialized it, highlights Michèlle Simondon (1984). The memorial is not identified with the monument and is not limited to it: it is usual to set the fragility of the monument against the eternity of the poem. Ancient Greece celebrates Mnemosyne through its poets (Hesiod, Pindar, and Euripides) and its works of art. The Greeks made memory an obligation, a duty, a moral value. But in addition to the function of revelation and immortalization, the Greeks granted another power to Mnemosyne (goddess of memory): that of transforming memory into the power of forgetting. Naturally, not just any forgetting. The form of forgetfulness

* Modified version of an article published in Spanish in the *Revista de Psicoanálisis* , Vol. 59, No. 2, April–June 2002 (published by the Argentine Psychoanalytic Association); and in the *Revista de Psicanálise da Sociedade Psicanalítica de Porto Alegre*, Vol. 16, April 2009.

DOI: 10.4324/9781032647791-24

advocated by Mnemosine is beneficial and creative, necessary for the functioning of memory. As D. Maronitis writes (quoted by Simondon, 1984): "here oblivion is no longer the enemy of poetic memory, but in a certain way its prologue and epilogue. The functioning of poetic memory begins when the rapporteur and the auditors have forgotten their present and personal torments and opens their spirit to a more significant and more collective past." If the story begins with oblivion, its charm, in turn, provokes oblivion. The creative aspect of memory, its future strength, constitutes the most constant and original in the Greek tradition. But paradoxically memory, says Simondon, "to remain active and lively, must be loaded as little as possible with dead memory." The commemoration is not the celebration of the motionless time of the statues, but that of a time in continuous resignification and movement, highlighting the past, announcing the becoming.

Remember, forget, metapsychological plot

In a certain sense we could say that psychoanalysis was born dealing with memory and forgetting or, more precisely, with the requirement imposed on the psychic apparatus to keep thoughts, images, sensations, or affections, lived as intolerable for the subject's ego, away from consciousness, either because they are too painful or incompatible with the value system of the person. Freud, in his passage through the Salpêtrière, observes that, for the first time in the history of medicine, Charcot creates or suppresses bodily symptoms through an exclusively verbal procedure, hypnosis, during which memories arose, which were placed contemporaneously with the appearance of the symptom. It is known, to venture into the past and the hypnosis would be quickly abandoned by Freud in favor of so-called "free association." In "On the Psychical Mechanism of Hysterical Phenomena" (Freud, 1893, p. 28), which he wrote years later with Breuer, he postulated their traumatic origin. The psychic trauma, and then its memory, act as a foreign body that keeps the symptom active. The therapy consisted of remembering the scene that had motivated the triggering of the symptom. The symptom is a substitute that arises to remove from consciousness those desires that are in conflict with the person's beliefs or value systems. But they are forgotten only in appearance. The symptom testifies to the conflict between the desire to forget and the desire to remember. Freud and Breuer initially spoke of "double consciousness," to emphasize the existence of another place, of another scene, Lacan (1960, p. 813) will say later, where those psychic phenomena that the subject wished to keep out of consciousness were located. The neurotic, claimed Freud, suffers from reminiscences or, rather, from a lack of reminiscences. He/she is not cured except to the extent that he/she manages to recover the memory, freed in the actualization of the transferential relationship, of the concomitant affective charge. The psychic mechanism at play in this effort to forget will be censorship and the content of the apparently forgotten, the repressed. The subject will be divided between their consciousness and their unconscious, and repression, for Freud, becomes the "pillar on which rests the whole edifice of psychoanalysis" (1914b, p. 11). The traumatic experience, he will say later, redefining what he called "his neurotic," does not necessarily require for the trauma to have existed in the external reality of the subject, their own desires or thoughts can be traumatic, always occupying throughout their theoretical development sexuality, one of the poles of all conflict. In that sense we can say that the psychoanalytic experience would act as a traumatic experience, which to the extent that it is lived as sufficiently contained, it will offer the subject the possibility of moving from a compulsive memory to a memory with representative capacity. Repression, memory, and forgetfulness constitute a plot that is inextricably linked to the vicissitudes of the symbolic organization of thought and its sexual foundation. Since our libidinal organization conditions the course of our thinking, one could say that they think and eventually remember from their own drive.

In a brief article, "Fausse Reconnaissance (Déjà Raconté) in the Course of Psychoanalytic Work" (Freud, 1914a), with the mastery that characterizes it, Freud warns about the conviction that some patients may have of having already told a fact remembered by them (p. 203). These phenomena of paramnesia include *déjà vu* [already seen], *déjà entendu* [already heard], *déjà eprouvé* [already experienced], *déjà senti* [already felt], *déjà raconté* [already told]. They all have in common an unexecuted unconscious design. For example, having experienced death wishes with respect to someone close, desires that I had never made conscious until the moment when a fact appears that makes one conscious and of which I thought I had already spoken previously. It can also operate as a concealing memory, concealing memory that, when related, works as if it had also related the second memory that actually hides behind the first. For example, Freud relates that a patient (the Wolf Man) relates in the course of their associations: "When at the age of five I played in the garden with a knife and cut off my little finger—oh! I just thought I had cut it... . But I have already referred it to you." When Freud asserts that the Wolf Man had never told him anything like it, the patient was surprised. To avoid a useless polemic, he asks them to repeat history anyway.

> I was 5 years old; I played in the garden with my babysitter and cut with my razor the bark of one of those walnut trees.... Suddenly I noticed with unspeakable terror that I had severed the little finger of my hand, so that it only hung on the skin. I didn't feel pain, but I did feel great anguish. I didn't dare say anything; I crumbled on the bench immediately and sat there, unable to cast another glance at my finger. At last, I calmed down, looked at my finger, and then I saw that it was completely intact."

Freud's patient finally accepted that it was very difficult for them to have told that memory without Freud having remembered such proof of castration anguish in their childhood. The question then arises as to why they were so sure they had already told it. And then to both comes to mind another memory that had been told several times and with some insistence in the previous sessions: "Once my uncle was going on a trip, he asked my sister and me what we wanted. My sister asked for a book; I, a knife" (the knife that his uncle had brought them was, according to their recollection, the same one that appeared in the two stories). This last story had then functioned as a concealing memory of the repressed memory, as a substitute for the story about the supposed loss of the little finger (symbolic equivalent of the penis), a story intercepted by the resistance. In other words, remembering is not a simple activity, but a complex one. Not only can memories be more or less accurate, but even the most precise and intense can be at the service of resistance in the form of concealing memories. It is all the difference between the memory of photographs or computers—those barbaric machines only capable of reproductive memories—and human memories whose memory is always representative, creative, and eminently subjective, since it includes the logic of the ghost. Although in the particular case of photography, in terms of the reproduction of the real, and following Barthes (1980), it would be necessary to include the gaze of the photographer who makes a singular cut of reality. Traditionally there were disquisitions on the opposition between perception and memory: Is what we perceive a faithful copy of the thing, of the object that exists in the world? Is what we remember a faithful copy of what we perceive? In the same way as for Magritte the image of a pipe is not a pipe, an idea that he immortalized with his famous painting of a pipe and the inscription below it that says "this is not a pipe," a statement that left more than one perplexed; for psychoanalysis, memory is not a faithful copy of what we perceive. The memory of the thing is not the thing. As soon as we perceive an object, a situation, a person, its perception is related to countless perceptions and memories affectively associated with it that will make that perception a valid perception for that single person. We perceive and remember from a complex network of perceptions and memories of them, sifted by the affection, history, language, desire, and libidinal organization of each one.

In Letter 52 to Fliess, on 6 December 1896, Freud argues that " our psychic mechanism has been generated by successive stratification, for from time to time the pre-existing material of mnemic traces undergoes a rearrangement according to new nexus, a retranscription" (Freud, 1950 [1892–1899], p. 233), And later he adds: "Each subsequent rewriting inhibits the previous one and diverts the excitatory process from it." That is, memory is not static and immutable. It is dynamic and subject to successive reinterpretations. The past, from the psychoanalytic point of view, is not immutable, it has a future. I repeat Valery's phrase: "memory is the future of the past." The memory of it acquires different reliefs and meanings with the successive meanings that are made *a posteriori*. What characterizes the human psyche is, for psychoanalysis, the primacy of the *"après-coup,"* that is, of the resignification that each scene acquires later, as the memory is threaded with a complex system of meanings and metaphors that can change, for example in the course of an analytic process. Thought, says Claude Rolland (2006, p. 25),

> appears less as a psychic production, defined by a positive content, than as a movement of the apparatus of the soul: like an earthquake, it decomposes a certain organization of representations, to recompose them in another way or at another level, assigning it a form that is not reduced to a continent, but that helps the 'transubstantiation' of its content.

From psychoanalysis, memory is not an entelechy. For the human psyche we speak of remembering and not of memory, since remembering does not consist of a mere bringing to a present time a fact of the past, as when one requests the memory of the computer. In the act of remembering we are continuously recreating the remembered fact, in a recreation that will be modified with the symbolic network that the subject will weave. This conception moves away from classical neurology, which considered memory as essentially reconstructive, but not from contemporary neurobiology. Damasio (1994), in his book *Descartes' Error*, states:

> Images are not stored as facsimiles of things, events, words or phrases. The brain does not archive polaroid photographs. We have direct evidence that when we remember a certain object, a face, a scene, we do not achieve an exact reproduction of the original, but rather an interpretation, a new, reconstructed version. Also, as we go through years and our experience changes, the versions evolve."

This modern vision of neuroscience is in no way far from the psychoanalytic conception. In that sense we can say that Freud preceded many of the discoveries of contemporary neuroscience and was a pioneer in that field.

In "Remembering, Repeating, and Working-Through" (1914c), Freud summarizes what he proposes as the essence of psychoanalytic technique. In it he modifies in part the simple way of remembering that he had described at the beginning of psychoanalysis, while preserving as the basis of psychoanalytic treatment the need for remembering. Described in this article, another way of remembering is repetition. He states that the analyst "does not remember in general anything forgotten and repressed, but acts it. They do not reproduce it as a memory, but as an action; they repeat it, without knowing of course, that they do it" (p. 123). It is the actualization in transference that allows the psychic mechanism to be revealed.

This repetition in the transfer has the advantage in the best of cases of being able to be resumed in the framework of the session, thus taking the person to the path of memories, facilitating the way to overcome resistance by mediating a reworking of them. In other words, the repetition of certain choices that are summarized in acts is another way for the psyche to remember. And from this point of view one can say that the transferential link allows a reactualization of the primary affective experiences, and therefore it is also a way of remembering. More problematic is repetition outside the psychoanalytic context. From the 1920s, with the introduction of the death drive, Freud will take up the idea of repetition and, with the denomination of compulsion to repetition, he will put it under the domain of the death drive. The memory that is expressed through the compulsion to repeat is not a memory linked to symbolic representation. It could be said that it is a memory of inferior quality, since it maintains the blindness of the subject.

In one of his last works, "Constructions in Analysis" (1937, p. 257), Freud reminds us that analytic work consists in "recalling certain experiences, as well as the motions of affection provoked by it, which are for the moment forgotten in them. The symptom is the substitute for that forgotten." While it is clear that the work of the analyst consists in remembering "something experienced and repressed by them," Freud wonders what the work of the analyst consists of, insofar as from his place he cannot remember something that concerns the inner world of the analyst. His task, says Freud, is to "collect the forgotten from the signs that this has left behind; Rather, he has to build it" or, if you prefer, to rebuild it. Freud compares the work of the analyst to that of the archaeologist. Personally, I would say that it also resembles the work of the architect or the painter who restores a work of art. They try to give it its initial splendor, which does not prevent them from putting in brushstrokes that are their own, respecting the original style. It is the opposite of what they did in the Sistine Chapel, which in Italian is known as *"il braghetone."* The frescoes painted by Michelangelo were recently restored. One of the questions that arose was whether the work was restored according to the original, or whether the loincloths that the censorship of the church had added after the original painting in which the sex of the characters was seen were preserved. The Vatican preferred that the loincloths be preserved. The analyst's job, on the other hand, is to restore the initial work, without the cover-up of the denial.

In the same article Freud adds later: "he often fails to bring the patient to the memory of the repressed. Instead, if the analysis has been executed correctly, one attains in them a certain conviction about the truth of the construction, which in the therapeutic has the same effect as a recovered memory." Each construction we consider a hypothesis, a conjecture, waiting to be examined, confirmed, or dismissed. It will not necessarily bring back memories like a net catching fish, but it will provide a significant force capable of supplying the mnesic faults. That is to say that one does not necessarily seek a construction that possesses a historical truth, but that fulfills a function in the dynamics of the psychic apparatus. And Freud even proposes that the term reconstruction replace that of interpretation.

The way of remembering is different depending on the psychic structure of the subject; it is not remembered in the same way from hysteria, from an obsessive neurosis, from a fetishistic perversion, from a melancholy, or from a delirious or hallucinatory psychosis. That is to say that the significant chain of the subject determines the modality of recall. The subject does not have a history that an observer could unravel and describe, he is his history and artisan of it, given his activity of remembrance in which past, present, and future are recreated as times in mutual interaction. There is no serene memory; it is always subject to the pressure of and the influence of the superego, which orients towards the approval or censure of the memory. It is convenient to mourn an exact remembrance for the benefit of creative reconstruction.

On the other hand, as J.-B. Pontalis said when interviewed by Pierre Nora (1977): "there is not a single memory, not even for the individual. There is a narrative memory, a phantastic memory, a memory of the body, a memory of that which was lived too intensely to be sufficiently elaborated, and a memory of that which was not sufficiently lived to be forgotten." But in all of them, the most important thing is the posteriori resignification that constantly modifies from the present, the putting into perspective of the past. Micheline Enriquez (1987) says that in every human being who aspires to think of themselves as a singular individual there is a subjective insistence that pushes them to recall. Psychoanalysis is a work of words that have a symbolic efficacy through a work of memory on memory.

But it is convenient to differentiate what Enriquez calls the immemorial and unforgettable memory from the memorable and forgetful memory. The first is a memory that does not lie in the realm of the memorable. Although it resists the wear and tear of time, it is constituted by a varied set of extremely early impressions. This memory is not thinkable in terms of the past. While it belongs to the past, it remains partly or totally unknowable. Only a few clues allow us to deduce its existence. This memory is of unconscious input. It would not be reappropriable in the first person, but through what Enriquez calls the deductive imaginary of the analytic situation, which allows us to arrive at an analytic construction, thanks to the effectiveness of its figurative potential. Memorable and forgetful memory corresponds to the amnesia that occurs as a result of a psychic conflict, secondary to secondary repression. It is by definition unfaithful, always in transformation; it is written and re-inscribed in temporality, sometimes filtered by concealing memory. I think that every analytic construction presupposes a prior deconstruction. Memory is one thing, and remembering is another. It is not the immutable memory of the hypercalculia of the psychotic child that has a symbolic efficacy. To remember and resignify the past, you have to be willing to forget and remember simultaneously, to be able to deconstruct and reconstruct a new symbolic plot that allows you to unknot the symptom. To Mnemosina, goddess of memory, the Greeks opposed Letha—that is, death, which represented oblivion. From the psychoanalytic point of view, I would say that one cannot intervene without the other. In other words, the life drive needs the death drive to induce change. In order to create new psychic bonds—which characterizes the life drive—the psychic apparatus must be willing to detach—what characterizes the death drive—the previously established bonds that were responsible for the pathological state. In his "Note Upon the 'Mystic Writing-Pad'" (1925. p. 230), Freud compares the functioning of the psychic apparatus with this device that allows him to answer the question: How to reconcile the immobility of trace and forgetfulness and the possibility of non-saturation? The whiteboard offers not only

> a receptive surface always usable, but also durable traces of characters, such as plain paper; It solves the problem of bringing both operations together by distributing them into two separate components—systems—which are linked together. That is exactly the way in which our psychic apparatus processes the function of perception. The stimulus-receiving stratum—the *P-Cs* system—does not form lasting footprints; the bases of remembrance take place in other, contiguous systems."

But memory is not an independent entity, independent of repression. As Gantheret (1977) emphasizes, memory in Freud's work participates in the very operation of repression. In the hypothetical case that this might not happen, we have "Funes el Memorioso," a famous story by Borges (1944). Borgean fiction consists of imagining that after having fallen from a horse, Ireneo Funes was crippled and suffering from hypermnesia. "Two or three times I had rebuilt a whole day; I had never hesitated, but each reconstruction had required a whole day." Until the day of his accident, says Borges, he had been what all humans are: "a blind man, a deaf, a bulge, a forgetful."

Borges (1944, p. 489) says that

> Locke, in the seventeenth century, postulated (and disapproved) an impossible language in which each individual thing, each stone, each bird and each branch had its own name; Funes once projected an analogous language, but he undid it because it seemed too general, too ambiguous. Indeed, Funes not only remembered every leaf on every tree on every mountain, but every time he had perceived or imagined it. Not only did he find it difficult to understand that the generic dog symbol encompassed so many disparate individuals of various sizes and shapes; It bothered him that the dog at three and fourteen (seen

in profile) had the same name as the dog at quarter past three (seen from the front). His own face in the mirror, his own hands, surprised him every time.

We all keep in mind that to be able to be aware of our identity, it is necessary to have a certain degree of memory. In the absence of it, someone could go to bed as if called Peter and wake up the next day believing it to be Paul. But the interesting thing about Borges' story is to draw our attention to something of which we are, it seems to me, less aware, and that is that in order to preserve the feeling of identity, we must also be able to forget. Otherwise, what happened to Funes would happen that not only was he surprised every time he looked in the mirror, believing that he was someone else, but he was also unable to think. Constructive forgetfulness—unlike denial, cleavage, or forclusion—allows a free circulation of representation within the psyche. It would be a form of forgetfulness in the Greek sense of the term: to free oneself from a dead, viscous, immutable memory, which prevents the creation of new significant links.

Psychoanalysis is a tool for re-appropriating its history by the subject, thanks to the updating of it in transference. A memory that escapes consciousness rests on transgenerational bases and is nourished by previous generations. As Michel Neyraut (1997) says, psychoanalysis uses the memory of the past to create a future that is not just repetition. The psychic apparatus functions as a conflicting alchemy of remembering and forgetting. But the two elements of that alchemy are necessary to maintain the sense of identity and the ability to think and also the perpetual balance between the imagination of memory and the creative capacity of forgetting.

I remember and forget, I build–deconstruct–rebuild, therefore I am.

References

Barthes, R. (1980). *La chambre claire*. Paris: Gallimard.

Borges, J. L. (1944). Funes el Memorioso. In: *Ficciones. Obras completas* (pp. 485–490). Buenos Aires: Emecé, 1974.

Damasio, A. (1994). *El error de Descartes. La razón de las emociones*. Santiago de Chile: Andrés Bello, 1996.

Enriquez, M. (1987). L'enveloppe de mémoire et ses trous. In: *Les enveloppes psychiques* (pp. 84–95). Paris: Dunod.

Freud, S. (with Breuer, J.) (1893). On the psychical mechanism of hysterical phenomena: A lecture. In: *Standard Edition, Vol. 3*. London: Hogarth Press, 1962.

Freud, S. (1914a). Fausse reconnaissance (déjà raconté) in psycho-analytic treatement. In: *Standard Edition, Vol. 13*. London: Hogarth Press, 1962.

Freud, S. (1914b). On the history of the psycho-analytic movement. In: *Standard Edition, Vol. 14*. London: Hogarth Press, 1962.

Freud, S. (1914c). Remembering, repeating and working-through. In: *Standard Edition, Vol. 12*. London: Hogarth Press, 1962.

Freud, S. (1925). A note upon the "mystic writing-pad". In: *Standard Edition, Vol. 19.* London: Hogarth Press, 1962.

Freud, S. (1937). Constructions in analysis. In: *Standard Edition, Vol. 23.* London: Hogarth Press, 1962.

Freud, S. (1950 [1892–1899]). Extracts from the Fliess Papers. In: *Standard Edition, Vol. 1.* London: Hogarth Press, 1966.

Gantheret, F. (1977). Trois mémoires. *Nouvelle Revue de Psychanalyse, 15*: 81–92.

Lacan, J. (1960). Subversion du sujet et dialectique du désir. In: *Écrits.* Paris: Seuil, 1966.

Neyraut, M. (1997). La mémoire inconsciente comme limite épistémologique. *Revue Française de Psychanalyse, 80* (No. 2, 2016): 125–136.

Nora, P. (1977). Mémoires de l'historien, mémoire de l'histoire. In: C. Couvreur et al. (Eds.), *Psychanalyse, neurosciences, cognitivismes* (pp. 43–50). Paris: PUF.

Rolland, J.-C. (2006). *Avant d'être celui qui parle.* Paris: Gallimard.

Simondon, M. (1984). La mémoire chez les anciens grecs. In: *Corps écrit* (pp. 51–64). Paris: PUF.

Index

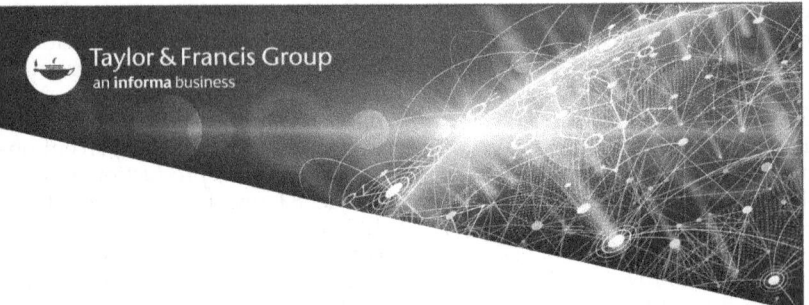
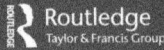
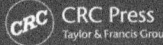